OH GOD!

ALSO BY SUSAN NEWMAN

*With Heart and Hand: The Black Church Working
to Save Black Children*

OH GOD!

A Black Woman's Guide to
Sex and Spirituality

THE REVEREND DR. SUSAN NEWMAN

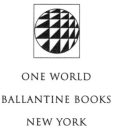

ONE WORLD

BALLANTINE BOOKS

NEW YORK

To my parents,
King Milton Newman
and
Lillian Dabney Newman

With love, "The Baby."

Contents

ACKNOWLEDGMENTS

First and foremost, I want to thank God for walking with me, until, at the age of thirteen, I decided to walk with God. I thank my mother, whose prayers, love, and tears have always sustained me. I thank my sister, Connie, who gave me pink bunny-rabbit flip-flops that I've worn during this whole writing process, as a reminder that she has always known the *real* me.

I thank my editor, Anita Diggs, and the Random House/Ballantine staff. Much gratitude to my agent, Djana Pearson-Morris, who saw in my writings what I didn't see. Blessings go out to TaRessa Stovall, who provided me shelter when I was in a storm (I'm still not drinking soy milk!). Thank you to my readers Lori Robinson, Mary Tilghman, Mark Toor, and Joye Brown Toor.

Special love to the members of the Mary and Martha Women's Bible Class, at the First Baptist Church (Randolph Street), in Washington, D.C. These mature, highly seasoned, and spicy women opened their hearts and minds to my teaching about being God's women. Thank you to every church in which I've served as pastor or associate pastor. Whether our time together was warm and fuzzy or wet and soggy, God was in all of it, working it for our good. Much love to Mt. Sinai Baptist, Zion Baptist, Peoples Congregational United Church of Christ (love you, Tony), Shiloh Baptist, and First Baptist, all of D.C.; St. Paul Baptist in Maryland; West Oakland Missionary Baptist, First Congregational United Church of Christ, and Rush Memorial United Church of Christ, of Atlanta, Georgia.

Thank you to the Jones family—Alan, Sharee, Calida, and Jonathan; the Frank Davis Sr. family (all one hundred of them). To Dr. Edward L. Wheeler, a wonderful friend who constantly encourages me to stretch forth. Gratitude to Dr. Flora Bryant, for answering my questions about clinical therapy. Heartfelt gratitude to the staff of the Extended StayAmerica Hotel in Landover, Maryland, especially Misché, who was gracious to me during the two months I stayed there writing. Words are not sufficient to express my love and gratitude to Rev. Benjamin L. Reynolds and the members of Emmanuel Baptist Church in Colorado Springs, Colorado. Let's just say . . . "You know!"

Thank you to the men who have been fathers, friends, brothers, and lovers. Special love to the ones who had my back in the slim times, Father Rob Wright, Dr. Wyatt T. Walker, Dr. Tim Winters, Dr. Robert J. Williams Sr., Rev. Johnny R. Johnson, Rev. Joseph Johnson, Rev. Peter Matthews, Dr. Rubin Tendai, LTC, Dwayne O. Hill, Alan Jones, Al Davis, and Donald Mann. My heart is always open to ViZion, a brother beloved, who helps me see new things whenever we're together. Thank you, my special friend, who surprised me with your love and reminded me of the joys in life's simple pleasures.

ACKNOWLEDGMENTS

Love and kisses to my SisterFriends, Joye, TaRessa, Dr. Yvonne Wilson, Djana, Nikki Mitchell, Tamara Nash, Michelle Collison, Dr. Kelly Brown Douglas, Lynell Green, Rev. Barbara Latoison, Rev. Countess Clark, Brenda Miller, Lori Robinson, Kelly Peterson, Catherine Foster, Marcell Johnson, Malinda Michael, Kathy Stanley, Rita Morgan (the Georgians) and Tina Blackwell (keep the umbrella up).

Most important, I want to thank my spiritual teachers, Deaconess Clara Powell, of Goodwill Baptist Church, and Rev. Mary E. Tilghman, Pastor of the Agape Bible Fellowship. Deaconess Powell showed the love of God in her life and upon her face. From the time I was eight years old, she took time to nurture me spiritually each week in Sunday school. I could see Jesus in her life and words. In November 1970, during youth revival at Goodwill, it was through the preaching of a guest evangelist, Rev. Tilghman, that I accepted Jesus Christ as my Savior at the age of thirteen. The following Sunday I was scheduled to be baptized. It was Deaconess Powell who helped me dress in my baptismal gown, as she sang hymns and prayed with me. For the next three years, I attended Rev. Tilghman's Bible class every Thursday night. If any of us missed class, Mary would call us before we left for school on Friday morning, asking, "Daughter, why weren't you in class last night?" In the 1980s, as an ordained minister, I was blessed to eulogize Deaconess Powell one Christmas Eve. Mary Tilghman and I have remained dear friends to this day. The Holy Spirit in the lives of women is an awesome thing to experience. Thank you, Lord!

Author's Note

Two versions of the Bible are quoted throughout *Oh God!* When the King James Version is quoted, "(KJV)" follows the text. All other quotes are taken from the New Revised Standard Version.

INTRODUCTION

Do you think I really wanted to write this book? Not hardly. I've done just fine for the last twenty-five years preaching, teaching, consulting, executive directing, and being my wonderful, God-called, Jesus-inspired, and Holy Ghost–anointed self. However, the topic of sex and spirit has always fascinated me. They seemed like flip sides of the same coin, and the name of the Lord is called upon in moments of ecstasy in both arenas. I've had my own personal opinions about the role of sex in our society and especially in the lives of black women and the Black church. But, with the exception of a few close friends, I've kept my opinions to myself, at least until *The Washington Post* exposed me.

In July 2000, I participated in the National Black Religious

Summit on Sexuality as a facilitator for a workshop on sex as a taboo subject in the Black church. I was not the speaker, just the facilitator. After the lecturer finished speaking, I facilitated the Q & A session; you know, I pointed at someone when it was her turn to ask a question of our lecturer. Everything was going fine until a woman said, "I don't see what sex has to do with the Black church at all!" Well, I couldn't keep quiet any longer. I shared an analogy that my former seminary professor, Dr. Harold Hunt, had shared with our class about how worship in the Black church was similar to a man and woman making love—in its passion and in the gradual crescendo in pitch and fervor. Of course, the reporter present attributed this analogy to me, rather than to Dr. Hunt. On Saturday, July 22, 2000, I was eating breakfast and reading *The Washington Post*'s Religion Section. I turned the page and there in 5,000-point type was the six-column headline: SEX, SINS, AND SERMONS. The whole page was an article about the summit, and there was a banner quote from me along with the analogy, attributed to *me*.

I was ready to call my travel agent and book a one-way ticket to the Bermuda Triangle! I could not believe this was happening. My opinions about the Black church, women, and sex were now available for all the readers of *The Washington Post*, which has a circulation of gazillions.

But all of this let me know that I had to write *Oh God!* Somebody has to own up to the fact that black folks need to start talking about sex from the sphere of the church. All of black life has its origins in the church, and we need to not let sex stand outside of our sanctuaries as if in punishment. The schools teach about it, the news media talk about it, the magazines write about it, the movies screenplay it, the stage dramatizes it, our musicians sing about it, our poets prose about it, the hip-hop generation raps about it, but we sit silent, as if we only praise the Lord under the sheets at night.

I want to talk about sex and black women. Don't get me wrong, I love men, but I have to start within my own context as a black woman of faith and spirit. I want to talk about what I've seen, what I've heard, what I know. There is much that needs to be said, and I guess I'll just start the frank, honest conversation. I'm not talking about sex, as we have traditionally understood it in the past. I'm not talking about how we wish sex would be in the future, I'm talking about what is the true and honest presence of sex in the lives of women today, right now.

I don't want to talk to your pastor, your girlfriend, your coworker; I want to talk to *you*. Yes, you. The one who is holding this book right this minute. Do you think it is an accident that we are having this conversation? I don't think so; there are no accidents with God, only providence. It would be easy to reiterate what has for years been taught and held up by churches, communities, and families, but that's not what women are wrestling with daily. Let's talk about what is truly going on in women's sex lives. Some women are married, and they enjoy good sex with their husbands. Some women are married, and when it comes to sex, well, let's just say they'd rather watch paint dry. Some women who are widowed or divorced have a companion with whom they are sexually intimate, but because of their religious teachings they feel guilty about it. Some women are single and never intend to marry, and some are single and are on a mission to find a mate. Some are having sex and enjoying it, or having sex and feeling guilty afterward. Others are either abstaining from sex and hating it, or abstaining from sex and enjoying their celibacy. In which category do you fall? No matter what your category is, *Oh God!* can help you have healthier, more balanced, and fiercely honest conversations with yourself and your God about sex.

If you are looking for a list of loopholes in the sexual codes of the Bible, you won't find any—there are none. The culture, traditions, and laws pertaining to Hebrew women and the moral code in an ancient civilization are *entirely* different from those pertaining to women living in this century. Women today, except in some Middle Eastern countries, are not the property of their father, husband, or nearest male relative. Women are wonderful human beings, created in the image of God. They live today as individual people who work in and outside of the home. They are married and single. Some are mothers and some are not. Women have made great contributions to our culture and society, but in spite of all their achievements in every area of life, when it comes to issues of sex and sexuality, there is still a double moral standard for men and women. Our church and society still hold women to a greater restriction, based upon gender. The last frontier of freedom for women today is a sexual one. This book in no way is the final word on the subject of sex and spirituality, but it is the beginning of the conversation for the Black church. Women can decide for themselves how to live natural, healthy, sane, spiritually powerful lives based on their love for God, self, and neighbor. These same women, after wrestling with their own demons and being delivered from any oppression that may have afflicted them in the past, can be great agents for healing and love, after they themselves have been healed and affirmed by the power of God's love. It is then, and only then, that we can effectively teach our children to embrace their spirituality and sexuality with self-respect and responsibility. Our children can receive their education about sex from someone who knows that sex is a gift from God.

While conducting trainings on "How to Talk to Your Youth About Sex," I realized that many women could not talk about sex with their children because they had not had an honest conversation with themselves. We don't talk honestly about how we feel about sex. We repeat what we've been taught, rather than process our own thoughts and feelings. We're not honest about sex. We cannot even use the appropriate words for having sexual intercourse. We say "they slept together," rather than "they had sex and then fell asleep."

As adults we cannot teach our youth about being responsible in every area of their lives, especially sex, unless we talk about how we can be responsible. Of course, abstinence is always our first line of education with children and youth when talking about sex. But we are discovering that alarming numbers of our youth are not abstinent; therefore, we need sex education curriculums that address the current mind-set of our youth and move them to a place of accountability. We have the opportunity today to educate our children about sex as a positive gift from God. As women of spirit, we can teach our children that their sexuality is a gift that they can experience with responsibility, when it is the most favorable time in their adult lives to do so.

So, with prayerful hearts and an open mind, let's have a new conversation about our sexuality and spirituality. It's always good to start at the beginning. Let's talk about what our parents told us about sex and how our thoughts about sex were formulated. Many of us received our initial religious training in Sunday school. We'll look at the Bible and rarely examined stories about Hebrew women and their lives in this ancient culture. We'll move on to look at Jesus Christ and his unique, nontraditional way of being with women and operating outside of the Jewish law to teach them. *Oh God!* will continue the conversation with a look at how black women as a collective body have been traumatized by slavery's lasting impression on our psyche.

This journey will be filled with tears and anger as we share in the horror of sexual abuse and domestic violence. But then there will be plenty of occasions to laugh out loud, too. All of this will culminate with a serious look at the possibilities for new and life-changing ministries in the Black church when it finally breaks its silence around issues of sex and sexuality. It is my desire that, at the end of this journey of challenge, reflection, education, and inspiration, you, my sisters of faith, will be able to covenant with your God in an honest, love-centered, and life-nurturing way, a new ethic to live by. This ethic will be your full expression of the greatest commandment to "love the Lord your God with all your heart, and with all your soul, and with all your mind, and love your neighbor as *yourself*."

Chapter One

The *Sexual* Truth Shall Set You Free

Can we talk? It is time for black women of faith to have an honest discussion about who we are sexually and spiritually. This generation of women must begin to confess that we love God, and we love sex, too! George Bernard Shaw said, "All great truths begin as blasphemies." Well, many in the church would call this statement blasphemous. But it is true. God created us with wonderful, healthy, natural drives—sleep, hunger, thirst, and sex—"and God saw that it was good."

On this journey of reconciling our sexual selves and our spiritual selves, we must be honest about who we are and what we desire, and we must learn how to live fuller, richer lives as spiritual women in the twenty-first century. Women who love God and are able to express themselves fully as sexual beings should be able to do so without shame or guilt.

Pam is a former party girl who accepted Jesus Christ as her Savior two years ago. She is a very attractive black woman who owns a home and earns a six-figure salary. Though active in her church and community, Pam is struggling with reconciling her sexual desires with the teachings of her faith. She wants answers to this dilemma. Is masturbation an acceptable sexual activity? Am I damned if I make love to my boyfriend because we are not married?

Donna is another woman of faith struggling with her sexual desires and the teachings of her church. Donna is forty-eight years old, widowed, and suddenly single again. After twenty-five years of marriage, the single life is foreign to her. She is confronted with a culture that includes HIV/AIDS, cybersex, Internet dating, and personal ads in the paper. She's too mature to go to clubs, but she doesn't want another husband. In the past, she had a wonderful marriage with the love of her life; now, she wants a companion and lover.

CHILDHOOD 101

Where do women get the idea that sex is wrong, that it should cause feelings of guilt and shame? When did we first learn about sex and how did we feel about it? A good place to start exploring answers to these questions is our childhood. I remember sitting in my fifth-grade class at John Quincy Adams Elementary School, in Washington, D.C., when the school nurse came in with an 8mm reel movie—it was time for our hygiene session. But today was different. She and the teacher had very somber, mournful expressions on their faces the entire time they set up the projector and screen. Watching them thread the film through the grooves on the projector reminded me of some ancient death ritual I'd seen on television. As the lights lowered and the movie began, we heard a serious male voice describing to us what our eyes could not believe. On the screen we saw diagrams of a man's penis and a woman's uterus and fallopian tubes. Then all of a sudden— without any of those "slasher movie" warnings—we were confronted with the image of the man's penis inside of the woman's vagina and thousands of sperm being catapulted into her body. Some of the kids in the room let out nervous laughter. Others sat there with our mouths open and our eyes bugging out of our heads. We were all shocked. Nothing could have prepared us for this scene. We sat there in the dark, watching millions of sperm swim into the vaginal canal and up the fallopian tubes, where one gold-medal swimmer united with an egg and rested in "the fertile lining of the woman's uterus." We sat in the dark, watching a bright movie screen as the words THE END stared back at us, a group of eleven-year-olds. The nurse gave the girls little pink booklets about menstruation and told us to refrain from sex so we would not get pregnant and have babies. The boys did not get anything, as if it were solely girls' responsibility to control the population of babies in the world. Go figure!

I went home that night knowing that what I had just witnessed in class was not true. I knew that my mother would tell me the truth about how girls got pregnant. Momma said, "When a boy and a girl are together, and they love each other, they have a baby." Well, Lawd have mercy, I was pregnant! I sat beside David Neverdon in class (we sat in alphabetical order), and I loved him.

My world had come to an end. I talked with the school nurse about the movie and what my momma had told me. She explained everything in greater detail to me. I then understood.

The next Sunday, as I sat in Sunday school, I looked at the superintendent and realized that he had three boys. My God! Mr. Green did that to Mrs. Green three times? Yuck! Nice Mr. Payne had eight kids! The pastor had five! I could not believe that these holy, sanctified members of the church performed that act I'd seen on the movie screen. However, I took pride in knowing that my parents did it only twice.

What were you told about sex as a child? Take a minute to think about it. Most sex education consisted of warnings like "Keep your legs together and your dress down," or "Don't bring no babies in this house!" I remember when my sister and I started going to house parties. Momma gave us several warnings. The warning I remember to this day is "When you're dancing slow with a boy, and he starts breathing hard—stop dancing!"

We were raised to fear sex and sexual expressions. When a girl began her period, it was as if there were a death in the family. She couldn't run and play with the boys anymore. An older woman in the family, usually the mother, brought out this secret, magic bag of mystery. The girl was instructed in "the ways of the Period." The bag contained the plastic-crotched panties, the elastic sanitary belt with loops (forerunner to today's thong), and finally the star of the show—the Kotex! It was a sanitary napkin, but it was more than an ordinary napkin. We called it "the Kotex!"

Every twenty-eight days we had to make a pilgrimage to the neighborhood drugstore to purchase the Kotex. God forbid if a male cashier should be behind the counter. We would read every last comic book and magazine in the store until he either went to lunch, went home, or just died. We were not going to purchase the Kotex from anyone but a woman. It was embarrassing. We felt shame just buying sanitary napkins. Isn't it funny that our husbands, brothers, fathers, and boyfriends are embarrassed to buy the Kotex, too? Well, that was sexual orientation 101—childhood.

As we matured from childhood to adolescence, our sexual orientation was filled with boys' pranks as they snapped our bra straps, looked under our dresses with mirrored shoes, and pushed us into the coat room with "that nasty boy."

SEXUAL ABUSE

While we are being honest about sexual truths, we cannot overlook the traumas that millions of women experience associated with sex. Unfortunately, for many women there are dark, scary, horrific experiences that are eternally bound to the sex act—incest, rape, domestic violence, sexual abuse. Many women are not comfortable with any sexual situation or relationship because of sexual abuse early in life. Some have found the courage to speak up about being sexually molested by teachers, relatives, babysitters, church leaders, or their own father. These were men whom they trusted as children, and their trust in any man was destroyed by the selfish, sick act of one man. Their minds are filled with the question: Was it something that I did to make him do this to me? Women who were victims in these situations blame themselves, as if it were their responsibility that they were abused. How can women who have been sexually traumatized as children embrace their own bodies and their natural sexual urges as good things? They were made to feel shame and guilt as children, and many still carry shame and guilt's offspring—unworthiness, fear, self-loathing, and depression.

Laura is a successful corporate executive. She's attractive, in her mid-forties, and the life of any party. She has been promoted within her company because of her business acumen. She is responsible for a staff of over 150 people and an annual budget of $2.5 million. But when Laura goes on a date and is faced with intimate situations, she becomes a frightened little girl. She may like the man she's out with, but she's not ready for any physical intimacy. However, she cannot say no to his sexual advances. She's a shark in the boardroom, but a guppy when alone with a man. It's as if she's in shock. It is like an out-of-body experience. She hears what he's saying, but she cannot speak; she knows what he's doing, but she doesn't possess the power to remove his hands. "If I say no, he won't like me anymore," and "It's my fault, I should not have worn this sexy dress," she reasons, giving in as though she has no choice.

THE RELIGIOUS *RIGHT*?

What causes sexual guilt and shame for Christian women? One source is the teachings of the apostle Paul. The teachings of the Christian church are based upon his teachings. Besides the four Gospels that include the life and teachings of Jesus, the majority of the New Testament consists of letters from Paul to various churches that he founded in ancient Rome, Ephesus, Philippi, Galatia, and Thessalonica. These places were under Roman rule and were greatly influenced by the Greek culture that was sweeping the world.

When interpreting the biblical text, we must look at the following: Who was writing the letter? To whom was it being written? What was the situation or problem that was being addressed? What was the culture of the day? Paul's advice to the church in I Corinthians 6:15–18 is:

"Know ye not that your bodies are the members of Christ? Shall I then take the members of Christ, and make them the members of a harlot? God forbid. What? Know ye not that he which is joined to an harlot is one body? For two, saith he, shall be one flesh. But he that is joined unto the Lord is one spirit. Flee fornication" (KJV). Fornication, in its original definition, comes from the Latin *fornicatus*, meaning to have intercourse with prostitutes or in a brothel. The word first appeared in 1552, during the same time frame when the King James Version of the Bible was being translated into English. In the sixteenth century, the Puritans of England were very troubled by the "loose morals" of the people and the booming business of the brothels in England. Some of the interpreters of the King James Version were Puritans.

Paul gives a lot of advice on sexual issues to this baby church in Corinth, a seaport city situated between Asia and Italy and the seat of commerce in the ancient world. Corinth was called "the eye of Greece," and it was there that various religions flourished alongside a small but growing cult of people—Christians. Sexual activity was a normal part of religious service, as seen in the worship of a hundred priestesses in the temple of the goddess Aphrodite.

Religious ceremonies were performed to ensure an abundance of food and the birth of children. The rites, expressed through dances, prayers, and incantations, symbolized the birth, death, and reappearance of vegetation, when acted out in a sacred drama. The fertility rite sought to control the otherwise unpredictable forces of nature. One of the main rites, concerned with increasing fertility of the land and the womb, was sexual orgies with temple prostitutes—hence, fornication. Many ancient fertility rites have persisted in modified forms into modern times. For example, the maypole dance derives from ancient spring rituals glorifying the phallus, or penis, with virgins (little girls) dancing around it with ribbons, celebrating the beginning of spring.

Paul, however, succeeded in stamping Christianity with a loathing of both sex and the body, from which we have never fully recovered. Early church fathers in the fourth century, in pious reaction to the excesses of Roman decadence, took to the North African deserts to become celibate, ascetic hermits of unbelievable strictness; this marked the beginning of monasteries and convents.

If one is going to interpret Paul's writings literally—and abide by *all* of his teachings—why not go all the way? In I Corinthians 7:6–8, Paul says, "But I speak this by permission, and not of commandment. For I would that all men were even as I myself. But every man hath his proper gift of God, one after this manner, and another after that. I say therefore to the unmarried and widows, it is good for them if they abide even as I" (KJV).

Stating a disclaimer, Paul admits that this is his opinion, not a commandment from God. Truth be told, like any preacher Paul gave instruction and advice to the early church filtered through a lens of his own values, prejudices, upbringing, and teachings. Paul was a Pharisee, a member of a Jewish sect that valued spirituality, ethics, and mysticism. They were the interpreters of the Jewish Law—the Torah. Paul was proud of his upbringing as a Jew.

If one is going to hold so firmly to Paul's advice about sex and relationships, then one shouldn't keep just part of Paul's instruction—one should keep it all! Consider, for example, Paul's Letter to Philemon. Paul told Onesimus, an escaped slave who converted to Christianity after meeting Paul, that he should return to his master, Philemon. Philemon was a Christian, so in his letter Paul appealed to Philemon's religious beliefs to not "be harsh" with Onesimus and to receive him back lovingly in servitude. Yeah, right!

Another instance of Paul's advice in a social situation is found in I Corinthians 14:33–35, which says, "For God is not the author of confusion, but of peace, as in all churches of the saints. Let your women keep silence in the churches: for it is not permitted unto them to speak; but they are commanded to be under obedience, as also saith the law. And if they will learn any thing, let them ask their husbands at home: for it is a shame for women to speak in the church" (KJV).

Well, in the early church, women sat on one side of the meeting room and men sat on the other side. For both sexes to mingle in public places was frowned upon. (Following this tradition, you wouldn't be able to sit next to your boyfriend at the movies anymore either!) When preachers would come and preach, making references to Jewish Law from the Torah, or Talmud or Midrash, the women would not understand the references and would cross the room to ask their male relatives. The men understood the references because Jewish boys studied the Torah and had a bar mitzvah (rite of passage into manhood). The boys sat with their fathers in the Court of the Men, near the altar of God, while the women sat in temple in the outer court, with the children and slaves. The playing field was not level for women in the early church.

The apostle Paul writes, "if they will learn anything," as if it were highly unlikely! Women were believed to be inferior to men. If a crime occurred in front of five hundred women, five hundred children, and one man, only the man would be allowed to testify in court. Such was the culture of the Jews in biblical times. Then Paul adds insult to injury, saying, "let them ask their husbands at home." Well, first of all (my hands are on my hips, and my neck is rolling) Paul assumes that every woman in church has a husband. Second, he thinks that when we get home from church, husbands want to sit down and debrief wives about the sermon? *Not!* I don't know about the men in your life, but after church on Sunday, it's either tip-off time, tee-off time, kick-off time, or time to eat and then take a nap. Few men want to have Bible study. Oh yes, Paul, how is a single woman going to learn anything without a husband to provide a debriefing?

So, if you are going to be a literalist when it comes to Paul's instructions, then, black women, forget about an orgasm, and just shut your mouths and go back to ole massa's plantation and pick a bale of cotton!

CULTURE, ART, AND MEDIA

Sex sells. When I was a little girl, I wanted to be the woman in the White Owl cigar commercial. She was a beautiful blonde who wore a seductive black dress. She was sexy, sultry, and attractive. Every man's eye was upon her—and I wanted to be like her. I also wanted to be the woman in the Noxema Medicated Comfort Shave commercial. She, too, was sexy. I never made it, though. I was seven years old, four feet five inches tall, and two feet wide, and my nickname was Butterball. My hair was dark brown and braided. I did not have a black, slinky, sexy dress. I wore clothes from the chubby department and black-and-white corrective shoes. So I got a cookie and forgot about that dream.

Sex in the media was subtle in the sixties, but we've come a long way, baby! I remember seeing the Frederick's of Hollywood catalogue, and it was something that you sneaked around the house to look at. I don't know why, because back then there was nothing sexy about a long-line bra with sixty hooks and a cross-your-heart-and-hope-to-die girdle. The underwear was made of industrial-strength rubber. Today, sex is in your face. The Victoria's Secret catalogue is as common in the mail as the phone bill. And the stuff in that catalogue is made of silk thread, a lot of hope, and air. If I put on one of those outfits . . . well, let's just say there would *be* no secrets.

Sex is on TV, in the movies, in music videos, in magazines, in newspapers, on the Internet. You ever have cybersex? Tell the truth, this is the "be honest" chapter of *Oh God!* Our culture has fooled you into having sex in front of a glowing box, with a total stranger, while typing with both hands. Don't laugh; some of you enjoy this and call it safe sex! I bless your choices . . . but I'd rather . . . never mind.

Music sends us sexual messages all the time. When a certain song is playing, I can be with a troll and fall madly in love, just because of the music. Tell the truth and shame the devil! God wants us to enjoy sex. If God did not want us to enjoy sex, She would not have made Barry White. If God did not want us to enjoy sex, He would not have made the Isley Brothers, Stevie Wonder, Smokey, Will Downing, the Dells, Harold Melvin and the Blue Notes with Teddy Pendergrass, Jeffrey Osborne with LTD, Luther, Marvin, D'Angelo, Maxwell, Lenny Kravitz, Prince, and R. Kelly. If God did not want us to enjoy sex, She would not have let us ever hear and slow drag to "Stay in My Corner," "Stairway to Heaven," "The Love We Had Stays on My Mind," "If Only for

One Night," "You Really Got a Hold on Me," "You and I," and "When Something Is Wrong with My Baby." Now, you go on and list *your* favorites.

_____   _____

_____   _____

_____   _____

Movies give out subtle and sometimes overt sexual messages about women and sexuality. In some movies, women are looked down upon or victimized. In November 1986, I saw Spike Lee's *She's Gotta Have It*. Nola Darling is a beautiful, assured sister, dating three very different men simultaneously: Jamie Overstreet—a controlling, protective, patriarchal type; Greer Childs—a wealthy, vain, arrogant male model; and Mars Blackmon—a comical, juvenile, immature jokester. Nola has gone beyond even a love "triangle"; but the stability of her love "square" is threatened by the increasing jealousy among her three suitors. Apparently, it was too much to expect Spike to portray Nola's character as an independent woman with a healthy sexual life throughout the movie. Jamie is determined to plant a flag in her back and make her submit to him. In the usual patriarchal form, he redeems this wanton woman by raping her into submission.

Strong, self-assured women are portrayed in movies as crazy—think about *Basic Instinct* and *Fatal Attraction*. Sexually active women are portrayed as prostitutes, loose, bad girls—consider *Set It Off*, Mae West, and Blaxploitation films. Asexual women are the mammies, full-figured, nurturing women. They are the matriarchs of the family—Ruth Younger in *A Raisin in the Sun*, and Big

Mamma in *Soul Food*. The movie culture really doesn't know what to do with lesbian women. Since lesbians do not want to be in an intimate or sexual relationship with a man, they are usually abused or killed, as in *The Women of Brewster Place*. Our media shows that a woman's desires and sexual expression have to be contained and controlled by a man.

As we got older the sexual messages from the world and culture was "do it," and the message from our parents was "don't do it." Our culture today is filled with booty call–type movies, strip clubs, and music videos in which all the women are wearing a thong and a bad attitude. Our young girls and boys are greatly influenced by these visual images.

PUPPY DOG *TALES*

I've always been puzzled by a ditty we learned as children that described the difference between boys and girls. "Sugar, spice and everything nice, that's what little girls are made of. Snakes, snails and puppy-dog tails, that's what little boys are made of." From childhood, we've had different expectations of boys and girls. Boys played with trucks and guns, and girls played with Barbie and Ken dolls. Boys were rough and aggressive. Girls were gentle and lady-like. A lot of things have changed since I was a child in the 1960s. Today, both girls and boys play Sony PlayStation and computer games. Girls participate in competitive sports like basketball and soccer, and they excel in martial arts and kick boxing.

However, many things have *not* changed. Our culture still sends out mixed messages about what is acceptable and expected from females versus males. Let's just look at the idea of marriage. Many women feel they have not completed their mission in life if they are not married. A lot of pressure is placed upon young women in regard to marriage. Some women have attended a family gathering only to have an aunt lift up their left hand and say, "No ring? Girl, you ain't getting any younger. All that education is fine, but you need a man." The men get the same kind of ribbing from well-intentioned aunts. "Raymond, you got a good job and money in the bank. It's time for you to settle down and start a family." At this point, the older men in the family rescue Raymond, saying, "Take your time, boy. You still got plenty of wild oats to sow."

Most women look forward to their wedding day. Our culture promotes it. There are several bride magazines that give advice about everything from choosing an engagement ring to planning a honeymoon. Women celebrate marriages. Men, on the other hand, are allergic to the very idea of marriage. When a couple announces their engagement to their friends and family, the women surround the bride-to-be with squeals of joy as they check out the ring. Meanwhile, the men in the room put their hands on her future husband's shoulders, shaking their heads, and sheepishly say, "Congratulations, man. I hope you're ready." For the woman, it's a new life. For the man, it's a life sentence.

Some of my funniest moments in ministry have been while performing weddings. The bride and her maids are in one area of the church, making last-minute beauty arrangements while laughing and sharing tears of joy. The groom is with me in my study, pacing back and forth, palms sweating, hands wringing, listening to his best man say, "I gotcha back, man. It ain't too late to change your mind."

The wedding day is the woman's day of delight and the man's day of dread. On the night before the wedding, the groom gathers with his buddies and has a bachelor party. The party usually features alcohol and scantily clad women prepared to perform lap dances and an array of other sexual favors for the groom in particular, and for the guests in general. It is expected that the groom will have his final fling before the wedding day. The purpose of the bachelor party is sexual pleasure for the groom.

The bride, on the other hand, has gathered with her female relatives and girlfriends for a bridal shower. They have plenty of food and punch. There's much laughter and teasing as the blushing bride-to-be excitedly opens her gifts, which are usually sexy lingerie to be worn during her honeymoon. The women teasingly tell her, "Girl, you'll blow his mind with this on." The purpose of the bridal shower is the ultimate sexual pleasure for the groom.

What's wrong with this picture? Women are expected to be virgins on their wedding night. Men are just expected to show up at the altar on time. Women spend their week before the wedding preparing to offer themselves to their husbands. Some men spend the night before the wedding sowing that last row of oats. Why are men not concerned about their virginity? No one at the wedding ever whispers, "I *know* he ain't wearing white."

Where did these unwritten rules and ridiculous expectations come from? Well, friends, they come from the Bible. Today is a new day. Knowledge is power, and as you learn more about yourself and the truth behind the Bible's messages about sex, you will gain the power to reconcile these two seemingly opposing forces in your life.

Sexual Affirmations

Starting today I will . . .

- be honest about my sexual feelings

- _____

- _____

- _____

- _____

Many spiritual women are not usually encouraged to look at their bodies in a positive way. Write what you feel is beautiful about your body. Include what you feel are your sexual attributes.

"I believe I am sexy because _____

_____

_____

_____

As you take this first step to sexual and spiritual reconciliation, reflect on where you are in your beliefs, and write a prayer of guidance for your journey:

_____

_____

_____

_____

Psalms 139:14 I will praise thee; for I am fearfully and wonderfully made: marvellous are thy works; and that my soul knoweth right well (KJV).

Quotables

"God is in me, with me, through me and for me.
Where God is, there can be no imperfection. Amen."

—DR. LEON WRIGHT, NEW TESTAMENT PROFESSOR, EMERITUS
HOWARD UNIVERSITY DIVINITY SCHOOL, WASHINGTON, D.C.

"I release the need to blame anyone, including myself. We are all doing the best we can with the understanding, knowledge, and awareness we have."

—LOUISE L. HAY

Chapter Two

What They Didn't Teach
You in Sunday School

I remember sitting in Sunday school reading the wonderful stories in the Bible. We were given little cards with colorful pictures depicting Jesus and a gathering of children or other scenes from the Bible stories. Sometimes the lesson would be about Jonah and the big fish, or God's deliverance of the Israelites from bondage in Egypt. From the beginner's class to the adult class, our Sunday school teachers never taught us how to distinguish between the spiritual value or lesson within a particular scripture and the cultural beliefs and traditions of the people portrayed in the scripture. It was never impressed upon us to sift through the passages and weed out the cultural traditions from the scripture's eternal lessons about love, justice, and grace.

Even as a young woman, I remember wondering why the lessons taught in Sunday school never had a woman as the main character. With the exception of the angel's visitation to Mary, the mother of Jesus, all women in our lessons were secondary or tertiary characters. When they did show up in Sunday school lessons or sermons, they were usually singled out for doing something negative. There was the usual citation of Eve, who yielded to the serpent and subsequently brought down the entire human race; Queen Jezebel, who brought idolatry to Israel; Rahab, the harlot; and we cannot forget Delilah and her deception of Samson.

None of the teachers or ministers of the church talked about the cultural traditions of women in the Bible. Many who teach in our churches today have not been taught the cultural, political, and social importance of the Hebrew people, whose lives and teachings we try to emulate.

Let's look a little deeper at the women in our Bibles. Women in ancient biblical times did not possess all the rights of a full person. They were the property of men—from the cradle to the grave. In Hebrew society women were subordinate, coming under the control of the father and passing from the father's dominance to the husband's. For example, the wife is listed along with the rest of the husband's property in the Ten Commandments, but not vice versa. "You shall not covet your neighbor's house; You shall not covet your neighbor's wife, or his male or female slave, or ox, or donkey, or anything that belongs to your neighbor" (Exodus 20:17). It was forbidden to covet a neighbor's wife but not a neighbor's husband; in this regard a wife was not a person, only a possession. In patriarchal days it was the husband's right, or at least the head of the family's right, to punish the adulterous woman (see Genesis 38:24, where Judah ordered Tamar burned).

The woman was not punished because she transgressed some sexual ethic but because, as property, she would jeopardize her husband's assuredness of paternity if she were to become pregnant. Lineage was a big thing in the ancient days. Remember reading all those begets in the Bible? It was the sole role of a Jewish wife to bear sons for her husband. If he died before she bore him a son, then she became the property of her dead husband's next male relative (usually a brother), and according to the Levite Law, she must bear a son with her brother-in-law in the name of her husband.

There was no punishment for the man who had sex unless he was caught doing so with a married or betrothed woman. In these cases of adultery, both the adulterer and the adulteress were to be executed: the adulterer because he had violated the property of another, and the adulteress for the reason noted above. Of course, since only the woman could become pregnant, she alone would be caught—and punished—much more often than would the man.

Most Christian women do not know fully how women are depicted in the Bible, nor of the relevance of their representation. We interpret our understanding of who we are as women of faith based upon the events in the Bible without any understanding of the culture or context of the scriptures. Usually when an issue confronts us, we ask, "What does the Word say about it?" We immediately go to the Bible and try to find a commandment or passage of scripture that deals with our concern, ignoring the fact that there are some differences from first-century Palestine to twenty-first-century America. It is important to understand who wrote the passage, when it was written, to whom it was written; aspects of the culture, customs, and traditions of the people at that time; and what was the particular situation that necessitated that response.

The picture of women revealed in the Bible is far from one-dimensional. The roles of biblical women range from concubine to queen, from prostitute to prophetess, from mother to murderer. Frequently subjected to the rule of their male counterparts, often adored because of their beauty, and occasionally praised for their leadership in time of crisis, women emerge from the pages of the Bible with as much complexity as the men. Women in biblical times lived in a patriarchal society. Both the Old and New Testament worlds normally restricted the role of women primarily to the sphere of home and family, although a few strong women emerged as leaders. We lift these sisters up on Women's Day at our churches—biblical women like Sarah, Ruth, Deborah, the Virtuous Woman of Proverbs 31, and others.

Children were almost totally at the disposal of the father, but daughters were so in a special way. Both daughters and sons could be sold into slavery, but after six years of service all male Hebrew slaves had to be freed by Hebrew masters. However, "when a man sells his daughter as a slave, she shall not go out as the male slaves do" (Exodus 21:7).

A more startling sexual discarding of daughters is found in the story of Lot and his daughters. Lot met two men on the road and invited them to spend the night at his house.

> But before they lay down, the men of the city, the men of Sodom, both young and old, all the people to the last man, surrounded the house; and they called to Lot, "Where are the men who came to you tonight? Bring them out to us, so that we may know them." Lot went out of the door to the men, shut the door after him, and said, "I beg you, my brothers, do not act so wickedly. Look, I have two daughters who have not known a man; let me

bring them out to you, and do to them as you please; only do nothing to these men, for they have come under the shelter of my roof" (Genesis 19:4–8).

A similar story occurs in the Book of Judges where the visiting man himself, a Levite (priest), shoves his concubine out the door to the mob to save himself. She is raped and beaten to death! A particularly distressing part of the story is that the Levite's concubine had run away from her "husband" back home to her father. After four months he went to fetch her and bring her back, and it was on the first night's journey back that she met her grim fate in Gibeah.

While they were enjoying themselves, the men of the city, a perverse lot, surrounded the house, and started pounding on the door. They said to the old man, the master of the house, "Bring out the man who came into your house, so that we may have intercourse with him." And the man, the master of the house, went out to them and said to them, "No, my brothers, do not act so wickedly. Since this man is my guest, do not do this vile thing. Here are my virgin daughter and his concubine; let me bring them out now. Ravish them and do whatever you want to them; but against this man do not do such a vile thing." But the men would not listen to him. So the man seized his concubine, and put her out to them. They wantonly raped her, and abused her all through the night until the morning. And as the dawn began to break, they let her go. As morning appeared, the woman came and fell down at the door of the man's house where her master was, until it was light. In the morning her master got up, opened the doors of the house, and when he went out to go on his way, there was his concubine lying at the door of the house, with her hands on the threshold. "Get up," he said to her, "we are going." But there was no answer. Then he put her on the donkey; and the man set out for his home. When he had entered his house, he took a knife, and grasping his concubine he cut her into twelve pieces, limb by limb, and sent her throughout all the territory of Israel (Judges 19:22–29).

The whole Hebrew tribe of Benjamin was severely punished. But nothing happened to, or is even said of, the Levite who shoved his concubine out to her death or the father who offered up his daughter to the same fate. Women were almost totally at the disposal of men in that society.

In the ancient biblical law, another instance of sexual immorality, where the woman was the victim of a double moral standard, is found in Deuteronomy 22:13–21. There, if a man claimed that his wife was not a virgin, the father of the bride was expected to bring out a garment with bloodstains resulting from the breaking of the hymen during her first marital intercourse and "spread out the cloth before the elders of the town." If the elders were satisfied, they fined the husband one hundred pieces of silver—payable to the father—and he would never be allowed to divorce the girl.

However, if the elders were not satisfied with the evidence, "They shall bring the young woman out to the entrance of her father's house and the men of her town shall stone her to death." The young bride, often less than a teenager, was in a no-win situation: If she lost her case, she was put to death; if she won, she had to live forever with a husband who was furious enough with her to try to have her killed, and was frustrated and had to pay a huge fine on her account. On the other hand, no man suffered a penalty for his lack of virginity!

If a husband suspected his wife of adultery or if he was jealous of her, he could force her to submit to an extremely humiliating and terrorizing trial by ordeal. This horrible experience is found in Numbers 5: 12–30.

> If any man's wife goes astray and is unfaithful to him, if a man has had intercourse with her but it is hidden from her husband, so that she is undetected though she has defiled herself, and there is no witness against her since she was not caught in the act; if a spirit of jealousy comes on him, and he is jealous of his wife who has defiled herself; or if a spirit of jealousy comes on him, and he is jealous of his wife, though she has not defiled herself; then the man shall bring his wife to the priest. . . . Then the priest shall bring her near, and set her before the Lord; the priest shall take holy water in an earthen vessel, and take some of the dust that is on the floor of the tabernacle and put it into the water. The priest shall set the woman before the Lord, dishevel the woman's hair, and place in her hands the grain offering of remembrance, which is the grain offering of jealousy. In his own hand the priest shall have the water of bitterness that brings the curse. Then the priest shall make her take an oath, saying, "If no man has lain with you, if you have not turned aside to uncleanness while under your husband's authority, be immune to this water of bitterness that brings the curse. But if you have gone astray while under your husband's authority, if you have defiled yourself and some man other than your hus-

band has had intercourse with you"—let the priest make the woman take the oath of the curse and say to the woman—"the Lord make you an execration and an oath among your people, when the Lord makes your uterus drop, your womb discharge; now may this water that brings the curse enter your bowels and make your womb discharge, your uterus drop!" And the woman shall say, "Amen. Amen." Then the priest shall put these curses in writing, and wash them off into the water of bitterness. He shall make the woman drink the water of bitterness that brings the curse, and the water that brings the curse shall enter her and cause bitter pain. The priest shall take the grain offering of jealousy out of the woman's hand, and shall elevate the grain offering before the Lord and bring it to the altar; and the priest shall take a handful of the grain offering, as its memorial portion, and turn it into smoke on the altar, and afterward shall make the woman drink the water. When he has made her drink the water, then, if she has defiled herself and has been unfaithful to her husband, the water that brings the curse shall enter into her and cause bitter pain, and her womb shall discharge, her uterus drop, and the woman shall become an execration among her people. But if the woman has not defiled herself and is clean, then she shall be immune and be able to conceive children. This is the law in cases of jealousy, when a wife, while under her husband's authority, goes astray and defiles herself, or when a spirit of jealousy comes on a man and he is jealous of his wife; then he shall set the woman before the Lord, and the priest shall apply this entire law to her. The man shall be free from iniquity, but the woman shall bear her iniquity.

I've counseled women who've experienced humiliation at the hand of their church because of the church's interpretation of various passages of Old Testament scripture. Jennifer Lewis, one of six children, grew up in rural North Carolina in the 1940s. Her father was a farmer, and her mother was a housewife. Her family attended Highpoint Baptist Church, where her father was a Sunday school teacher and her mother was a missionary. At the age of sixteen, Jennifer became pregnant. She was forced to come before the church, confess her sin, and plead for forgiveness. She stood before the deacon board and the ministers (all male) to receive her punishment. Jennifer was not allowed to play or associate with the other children in the church or community. She had to attend every church service and prayer meeting. When her baby was born, she was not allowed to have the baby blessed in the church sanctuary—the pastor came to the home and prayed for the child. The father of Jennifer's child was a nineteen-year-old who denied his involvement and joined the Marines.

Women have been robbed of the positive aspects of their sexuality in the Bible. And Christian women today are sexually frustrated because they have tried to literally interpret their lives today based on this ancient biblical text—but the women in the Bible simply are not us! Their lives were not the same as ours. They did not work in corporate America. They did not own their own property. They did not have the right to make choices about when to have children, how many to have, and what birth control method is available to them if they choose not to have children. These biblical women have great stories of faithful living in a culture that was oppressive to women. However, their culture does not translate to our culture. Their role and purpose in society is not the same as ours today. They are simply not us!

SEXUAL RESTRICTIONS ON HEBREW WOMEN

After the Jews returned to Jerusalem from exile in Babylon in the sixth century B.C., the men were instructed to drive away the non-Jewish wives and children they had acquired while living among the Babylonians (Nehemiah 13:23–28, Ezra 10:3). The prophets Nehemiah and Ezra strongly emphasized how important it was for this remnant of the Jewish people to develop an in-group defense as they returned to a land surrounded by people of different cultures and religions. They took drastic measures to retain group identity and unity. Jewish women were sexually restricted to ensure the purity and continuance of the Jewish male line. That's why polygamy (one man with many wives) was allowed, but polyandry (one woman with many husbands) was not.

After Alexander the Great's conquest of the area toward the end of the fourth century B.C. and the resulting spread of Greek culture, the restrictive Jewish attitude intensified even more. The Greek culture was so attractive and pervasive that the Jews saw it as a threat to their identity and way of life. They felt that they had to take steps to indoctrinate their community from its influences. Restrictions on women were increased to keep them separate from the Greek influences—especially their religions, which held women in higher regard than did Judaism. Hellenistic (Greek) religion and society included goddess worship. Well, the Jewish men did not want their women exposed to this, so they wrote rules that restricted how much a Hebrew woman could socialize outside of the home and her culture.

The early Christians were Jews who accepted Jesus as their Messiah. They believed the teachings of Jesus and accepted the gospel of Good News, but they still lived their daily lives in the old ways of their culture. A woman's social life was still very restricted, and the families and communities kept to themselves. In the beginning, Christians were looked upon as a cult or sect. They were a religious group of people with a charismatic leader. After their leader's death, their numbers grew, but they kept to themselves—"being separate from the world."

Christians in the first century A.D. were looked upon similarly to the way we view Amish people of today. The Amish have their own religious beliefs and social customs; they keep to themselves; and yet we peacefully coexist in the same country. Some Amish migrated to the United States in the early eighteenth century, settling in Pennsylvania, Illinois, Indiana, Iowa, Missouri, and Ohio. They have attempted to preserve the elements of late-seventeenth-century European rural culture, and they reject most of the developments of the modern society. Today's Amish probably total approximately one hundred thousand in twenty-two states, with about forty-five thousand in Ohio, and smaller numbers in Illinois, Indiana, Pennsylvania, and so forth. In addition, about fifteen hundred live in Ontario, Canada.

Formal education beyond the eighth grade is discouraged among the Amish. They do not use electricity, and they do not own or use automobiles, TVs, and radios. They do not take photographs because of the second of the Ten Commandments: "Thou shalt not make any graven image" (Exodus 20:4). The Amish's practices of not completing school beyond the eighth grade, not driving cars, not using electricity, etc., are not religious commandments, they are cultural traditions. The Amish have their own traditions today, just as Christians had their own traditions in the Greco-Roman world of the first century, when the New Testament was written.

We are doing a disservice to our daughters, and ourselves, trying to fit a 2001 peg into a 400 B.C. hole. We need to *change* the dialogue. We need to keep it real and tell it like it is. Women in ancient civilizations did not have to deal with sexual abstinence as women do today; girls were betrothed at the age of five and given in marriage between the ages of thirteen and sixteen. However, today we have women who go to college, pursue careers, and sometimes delay marriage and child bearing. There are some women who choose not to marry and have children. These women do not love God any less than a married woman with children. They are not any less spiritual, or any less righteous, because they have chosen a different path.

CHRISTIANITY'S FEAR AND LOATHING OF EROS

Patriarchal Christianity inculcated a fear of the body. The Greeks and Romans had a healthy love and adoration of both male and female bodies, as we see from their statues. As I mentioned earlier, there is no evidence that Jesus either looked down on women or abominated sex. If anything, he was sympathetic to women's inferior status and had very close women followers. The apostle Paul, however, had a different view. Paul was obsessed with preventing fornication. This was the chief value of marriage in his eyes. Though it was preferable by far to remain sublimely celibate like him, wherever the flesh is weak it is, in his immortal words, "better to marry than to burn" (I Corinthians 7:9 KJV)—the "burning" referred, of course, to lust of the flesh!

Paul and Saint Augustine (A.D. 354–430) succeeded in stamping Christianity and the West with a loathing of sex and the body, from which we have never fully recovered. "To Carthage I came, where there sang all around my ears a cauldron of unholy loves," wrote Augustine, describing the years of his temptations. Soon, following their lead, and in pious reaction to the excesses of Roman decadence, hundreds of men and women took to North African and other deserts to become ascetic hermits of unbelievable strictness.

Asceticism, from the Greek *askesis*, meaning exercise or training, can be found in all religions, but is more important in some, such as early Christianity. It typically involves celibacy, fasting, poverty, seclusion, and, often, a degree of self-mortification in a program of self-discipline and self-denial intended to achieve a spiritual goal, which varies from faith to faith. Within Christianity, ascetics had differing aims: some were divorcing themselves from the material world, some were performing penance, and others were attempting to share the sufferings of Christ.

The early fathers of the Christian church were not natural ascetics: they were men—often with active sex lives—tormented by their inability to control their desires. Saint Augustine prayed, "Give me chastity . . . but not yet." His contemporary, Saint Jerome, related how, when he was fasting in the desert, "I . . . fancied myself among bevies of girls. . . . My mind was burning with the cravings of desire, and the fires of lust flared up from my flesh that was as that of a corpse."

Jerome called sex unclean; the theologian and moralist Tertullian (A.D. 155–c. 225) called it shameful, and Saint Ambrose (A.D. 339–97) called it a defilement. For Augustine, it was specifically the loss of self-control that was so disturbing. Writing about the Garden of Eden, he exclaimed, "Perish the thought that there should have been any unregulated excitement, or any need to resist desire!" The very idea that one could have an appetite for sex, and enjoy it, was terrifying to Augustine. Procreation within marriage was the only acceptable goal of sex for him.

Penitential books (which list misdeeds and penalties from the sixth to ninth centuries) reveal that contraception was almost as sinful as murder, requiring penances that lasted from two to fifteen years. Even coitus interruptus (known today as the rhythm method)—the only form of contraception sanctioned by the Roman Catholic Church—was a sin, but it received lighter penalties than oral sex. The church also attempted to limit the days on which a married couple could try to procreate. Sex was made illegal on Sundays, Wednesdays, and Fridays; for forty days before Easter and Christmas; and for three days before communion.

Well, now, let's do the marital conjugal math: There are 365 days in a year, minus 52 Sundays, minus 52 Wednesdays, minus 52 Fridays, minus the 40 days before Easter, minus the 40 days before Christmas . . . so married couples are allowed to have sex how many times a year? Your guess is as good as mine! Sex is a gift from God, meant for enjoyment, not for regulation by abstinent monks.

THE SONG OF SOLOMON

There is one book of the Bible that church folk are more afraid of than the Book of Revelation, and that's the Song of Solomon, the most sensuous, sexual of all the books. Throughout history, there have been attempts to understand the Song of Solomon as an allegory. Some have viewed the Song of Solomon as a book about the love of God for Israel, but interpret the words as the love between a man and a woman. The Song of Solomon celebrates erotic love between a man and a woman in a mutually enjoyable friendship. The woman expresses her desires for her beloved as often as he expresses his dependency and expectation of her erotic love.

They praise the beauty and sensuousness of each other's bodies, and the book's eroticism is very descriptive:

My beloved is all radiant and ruddy, distinguished among ten thousand. His head is the finest gold; his locks are wavy, black as a raven. His eyes are like doves beside springs of water, bathed in milk, fitly set. His cheeks are like beds of spices, yielding fragrance. His lips are lilies, distilling liquid myrrh. His arms are rounded gold, set with jewels. His body is ivory work, encrusted with sapphires. His legs are alabaster columns, set upon bases of gold. His appearance is like Lebanon, choice as the cedars. His speech is most sweet, and he is altogether desirable. This is my beloved and this is my friend, O daughters of Jerusalem (Song 5:10–16).

How graceful are your feet in sandals, O queenly maiden! Your rounded thighs are like jewels, the work of a master hand. Your navel is a rounded bowl that never lacks mixed wine. Your belly is a heap of wheat, encircled with lilies. Your two breasts are like two fawns, twins of a gazelle. Your neck is like an ivory tower. Your eyes are pools in Heshbon, by the gate of Bath-rab'bim. Your nose is like a tower of Lebanon, overlooking Damascus. Your head crowns you like Carmel, and your flowing locks are like purple; a king is held captive in the tresses. How fair and pleasant you are, O loved one, delectable maiden! You are stately as a palm tree, and your breasts are like its clusters. I say I will climb the palm tree and lay hold of its branches. Oh, may your breasts be like clusters of the vine, and the scent of your breath like apples, and your kisses like the best wine that goes down smoothly, gliding over lips and teeth. I am my beloved's, and his desire is for me (Song 7:1–10).

Now I know why this is called the Song of Songs. Solomon is said to have written 1,005 songs (I Kings 4:32), and this is proba- bly the best one. These are but a few biblical passages that were never lifted up for critical review in Sunday school or Wednesday- night Bible study. A life application study of the Song of Solomon is not offered in the Christian Education Institutes of our churches. Neither have we been challenged to study critically the lives of women in the scriptures in light of their culture and beliefs ac- cording to the Hebrew Law. Well, there is one teacher who does not flinch at examining the Hebrew Law in relationship to women and all people—Jesus Christ.

How do you feel after reading about the Levite's concubine? Name ways in which some women today are still treated like the Levite's concubine or the woman subjected to the trial by ordeal.

_____

_____

_____

_____

The early church fathers called sex "unclean, shameful, and a defilement." What words do you use to describe sex in your life? Why?

_____

_____

_____

_____

In the Song of Solomon, the lover and the beloved describe each other in such wonderful ways. Think about your beloved, or someone you used to love, and write your own song of love.

"My Beloved's _____

_____

_____

_____

Now, write one describing yourself. "I am my Beloved . . ."

_____

_____

_____

Tell your beloved:

- What you truly feel
- Who you really are
- What you really want
- How to love you best
- How to listen to you

CHAPTER THREE

Jesus as the Liberating
Feminist of the Bible

Women in biblical times lived in an oppressive and unjust patriarchal society. Both the Old and New Testament worlds normally restricted the role of women primarily to the sphere of home and family, although a few strong women emerged as leaders. In religious life, women were subordinate to men. Fathers, husbands, and other male relatives gave protection and direction to women. But Jesus changed the conversation concerning women. He paid attention to them and acknowledged a woman's place in the Kingdom. His manner was inclusive, and He willingly went against the religious laws and customs of the Jews on behalf of women. By what Jesus did and what He said, he elevated the status of women.

Through his missionary journeys, Paul eventually realized the great contributions women could make in the work of the church. Although Paul saw the need to preserve order in the early church, he exclaimed in Galatians 3:28 "There is neither Jew nor Greek, there is neither bond nor free, there is neither male nor female; for ye are all one in Christ Jesus" (KJV). The final barrier preventing women from fully participating in the Kingdom of God toppled under Jesus' influence.

Jesus was able to retain the best in the Hebrew tradition and yet cut away some of the rigid structure that restricted it. He was able to do the same for women. Without radically changing their roles, Jesus enlarged and transformed women's possibilities for a full life. His manner and teachings elevated her status and gave her an identity and a cause. Jesus' manner in His instructions with women is at least as significant as His teachings about women. At the risk of censure from a male-oriented society, Jesus talked to women, responded to their touch, healed them, received their emotional and financial support, and used them as main characters in His stories. Women of that day could not be disciples or rabbis, but Jesus recognized women's potential for intelligent thought and commitment.

In Luke 10:38–42 there was an extraordinary incident recorded between Jesus and two sisters—Mary and Martha. Jesus was visiting the home of his three friends, Martha, Mary, and Lazarus. These three siblings offered Jesus their home in Bethany as a place of retreat and solace away from the critical eyes of the Pharisees and Scribes. One evening while Martha was in the kitchen performing the traditional acts of women—cooking, cleaning, and serving the meal—Mary was in the living room, *sitting at the Lord's feet,* which denotes being taught as a disciple. Martha was frustrated because she was doing the expected work and she wanted Jesus, in his role as the Jewish man, to reprimand Mary for not doing her expected womanly work. Instead of reprimanding Mary, Jesus reprimands Martha, saying, "Martha, Martha, you are worried and distracted by many things; there is need of only one thing. Mary has chosen the better part, which will not be taken away from her."

Besides seeing women as persons, Jesus involved them in His earthly ministry. Luke mentioned a group of women who traveled with Jesus as He journeyed from town to town (Luke 8:1–3). Among them were Mary Magdalene, Joanna, and Susanna. These women provided financial support for Jesus and the Twelve Apostles. Women also proclaimed the gospel. In His encounter with the Samaritan woman, Jesus revealed Himself as the Messiah. She immediately left and began telling people, "He told me everything I have ever done" (John 4:39). Many Samaritans believed in Jesus because of this woman's testimony. Women were the first at the tomb after the resurrection. As such, they were the first to broadcast His victory over death (Luke 23:55, 24:11). Matthew, Mark, and Luke all called attention to the loyal women who participated in Jesus' Galilean ministry and followed Him all the way to the cross and the grave. They received and shared the greatest news: "He is not here, but has risen" (Luke 24:5).

As a master teacher, Jesus used parables to teach about the Kingdom of God. He reached out to women in His audience by telling stories about their life experiences. In one trilogy of parables, Jesus depicts God as a shepherd whose sheep has gone astray, a father whose son is in a far country, and a woman who has lost her coin. As the woman who has lost one of her ten silver coins, God is depicted as lighting a lamp and sweeping the house until the coin is recovered (Luke 15:9, 10).

———

By capturing women's attention and commitment through parables, Jesus offered them a place in the Kingdom. Jesus' parable of the ten maidens, five foolish and five wise, hints at the way He saw and dealt with women (Matthew 25:1–13). He saw women as neither inferior nor superior, but simply as persons. He saw their potentials, sinfulness, and strengths, as well as their weaknesses. He dealt with them directly. He elevated their status as a group and strengthened their participation and influence in their world. As individuals, they were treated as friends and disciples. Women are the subject of many questions and controversies in the church today. Is she equal to a man? Can she exercise the same spiritual gifts as men in the church? Should she be subject to her husband in all matters? As Christians turn to the Bible for guidance in responding to these questions, they must be careful not to focus on one verse or passage. The *total* impact and message of the Bible should become the guiding spirit in answering these and other questions.

The Old Testament clearly subjected women to the will and protection of their husbands. They were celebrated for performing their important roles as wives and mothers, as seen in Proverbs 31:10–31. The question was asked, "Who can find a virtuous woman?" Then the writer of Proverbs goes on to list her virtues, which would spell burnout to any woman in any century. For the Hebrew man, he is known in the gates of the city by the tireless work of his wife. She cooks, cleans, weaves, sews, provides for her household and the households of others. She is wise in the marketplace. She works from sunup to sundown. She is admired for her physical strength and capabilities. Then, after praising her because of her hard work and sacrifice, the writer offers this virtuous woman a backhanded compliment, saying, "Charm is deceitful, and beauty is vain, but a woman who fears the Lord is to be praised." After reading this text for years, one day, while listening to it, I thought about our modern-day version of this woman. She works like a dog for her husband and children, who never say thank you, and when Mother's Day comes along, instead of getting a day at the spa as a gift, she is given a new vacuum or a washer and dryer.

On occasion, the Hebrew woman rose above her traditional role and led the Jewish nation in time of crisis. During the years when Israel had no king, she was led by nine Judges, one of them a woman—Deborah. In Judges, chapters four and five, the story is recorded of Israel's victory over Sisera through the leadership of Deborah, a prophetess of Lappidoth. Barak, the commander of Israel's army, did not want to go into battle unless Deborah went with him. She agreed, but warned him that the victory and honor would be given "into the hands of a woman."

The New Testament brings a different picture of women into focus. Jesus, and later Paul, elevated the status of woman so that she could be a full participant in the Kingdom of God. She is urged to use her responsibility as well as her freedom to find her place in the body of Christ. The spirit of freedom and the love in Christ belong to women as well as men.

Women witnessed Jesus' crucifixion, up close. Women, who had known His healing power, gathered at Jesus' feet in His finest and final hour. Motivated by gratitude, courage, and love, these women did not run away, hide, or deny Christ. In spite of His public humiliation and grotesque execution, these women wanted to be near this One who had done so much for them. Little did they know that their faithfulness would allow them not only to be eyewitnesses of Jesus' death, but also to be messengers of His resurrection, proclaiming He is risen!

GOD WITH US

Jesus was human and divine. I find it interesting that God thought so much of us that He would become one of us. Yet, we are constantly trying to deny our humanity. We try on numerous occasions, almost to the point of obsession, to "deny our flesh." But it was Emmanuel, God with us in the flesh, that brought wonder, miracles, light, and love into our world, and eventually into our lives. "Behold, a virgin shall be with child, and shall bring forth a son, and they shall call his name Emmanuel, which being interpreted is, God with us" (Matthew 1:23 KJV). If the God of Jesus Christ can live inside of this flesh, don't you think it's time we should embrace our own selves?

Let's look at Jesus.

He was a very sensuous man—earthy, good-natured, compassionate, and attractive. Yes, I said attractive. Think about it. Jesus walked everywhere he went, so he was in good cardiovascular health. He got lots of fresh air under the African sun. This sun-kissed Savior ate and drank with sinners and friends (who could be the same people). Children loved him, men admired him, women wanted to be near him. He nurtured his spiritual life by prayer and devotion. Early in the morning the disciples could find Jesus off alone somewhere, in prayer. His days were spent showing compassion to the people on the margin of society—people whom the rigid religious leaders would not think about speaking to, unless it was to utter a word of condemnation. Speaking of these religious leaders, one day, Jesus said, "That except your righteousness [code of ethics] shall exceed the righteousness of the scribes and Pharisees, ye shall in no case enter the Kingdom of Heaven" (Matthew 5:20 KJV). Throughout Jesus' three-year public ministry, the scribes and Pharisees observed Him, criticizing His lifestyle, teachings, and actions. They were waiting to catch Him breaking just one of the laws of the Torah.

The Gospel of John, chapter 8, records the story of the woman caught in the act of adultery. This story shows the insensitive use of a woman by a group of Scribes and Pharisees, who employ her to set a legal trap for Jesus. These men would go to any extreme to capture Him, this maverick of a rabbi, breaking the Law of Moses. First, the woman was surprised in the intimate act of sexual intercourse with an unidentified person. (According to Deuteronomy 19:15, there had to be two or more witnesses other than the husband, and they had to be male.) Unless the Scribes and the Pharisees were themselves the witnesses, it would seem that the poor woman was dragged before them, and that they, perhaps along with the witnesses, were dragging her to the Sanhedrin. Since Jesus was teaching in the area of the Temple at the time, the Scribes and the Pharisees apparently took the opportunity to use the woman to trap Him.

I believe, along with some of my theological colleagues, that the Scribes and Pharisees arranged this setup extraordinaire for Jesus. The situation presented Jesus with a dilemma. Here was a woman caught in the very act of adultery, and according to the Law of Moses, she should be stoned to death. However, Jerusalem was under the governmental authority of Rome, and citizens could not perform acts of capital punishment without a trial and decree from Rome. Thus, Jesus was faced with a catch-22. If He said, "Stone her," He would be in trouble with Rome. But if He said, "Don't stone her," He would be in trouble with the Scribes and Pharisees for not keeping the Law of Moses.

Can't you just see them, standing there with their religious robes full of rocks, ready for a good ole stoning? But what does Jesus do? How does this revolutionary feminist handle this situation? He chooses to not decide. Jesus puts the decision back on the angry mob of men gathered around this naked woman standing in the dust. Putting Jesus' words in today's vernacular, I can hear Him saying, "You're right, boys! Today is a good day for a stoning, but let me first lay the ground rules. The one brother out there in the crowd who is without sin, the one who has never cheated on his wife, never thought an unholy thought, never deceived anyone in business, that one brother can throw the first stone, and the rest of you righteous ones can join him." Though Jesus refused to get caught up in their legalisms, He dealt with their human nature. They probably would not have conceived of this scenario to catch Jesus if He had not already had a reputation for defending women.

It was obvious that this woman was guilty of the crime of adultery, since she was caught in the act. But where was the adulterer? No one commits adultery alone. According to the Law of Moses, the woman *and* the man were to be punished:

If a man is caught lying with the wife of another man, both of them shall die, the man who lay with the woman as well as the woman. So you shall purge the evil from Israel. If there is a young woman, a virgin already engaged to be married, and a man meets her in the town and lies with her, you shall bring both of them to the gate of that town and stone them to death, the young woman because she did not cry for help in the town and the man because he violated his neighbor's wife. So you shall purge the evil from your midst. But if the man meets the engaged woman in the open country, and the man seizes her and lies with her, then only the man who lay with her shall die. You shall do nothing to the young woman; the young woman has not committed an offense punishable by death, because this case is like that of someone who attacks and murders a neighbor. Since he found her in the open country, the engaged woman may have cried for help, but there was no one to rescue her (Deuteronomy 22:22–27).

Jesus touched people who were seen as "unclean" by society. He talked to lepers, who were ostracized by the people. Because they had an infectious disease that had no cure, lepers lived in caves and isolated areas away from society. They lived alone, their bodies in constant decay; their skin had lesions, their wounds were wrapped with bandages, some lost their nose and limbs. They were treated in ancient times the way some people treat those living with AIDS today. But Jesus loved the lepers; one day, when ten lepers approached him, seeking food or drink, Jesus fulfilled a greater need. He healed them and sent them to the Jerusalem board of health to be declared clean. Even though only one of the ten thanked Jesus, He showed compassion to all ten. Unconditional love is very attractive in a person.

Jesus showed compassion for women and healed them, too. Jesus saw women first as persons with both physical needs and spiritual faith, which, combined, got his attention. There is no record in the Bible of a Jewish woman requesting healing from Jesus, probably because Jewish women were conditioned by their culture to assume that a public religious leader would not recognize them.

It is important to note that in the Gospel of Mark, the first gospel written, Jesus begins his public ministry by healing a woman, Simon's mother-in-law:

> As soon as they left the synagogue, they entered the house of Simon and Andrew, with James and John. Now Simon's mother-in-law was in bed with a fever, and they told him about her at once. He came and took her by the hand and lifted her up. Then the fever left her, and she began to serve them (Mark 1:29–31).

One day, Jesus healed a woman who had been suffering with a constant menstrual blood flow for twelve years, a condition today called menorrhagia. This woman did not want to draw attention to herself, but she wanted to be healed, and she believed Jesus had the power to heal her. As a woman experiencing blood flow, she had been ritually unclean, according to Jewish Law (see Leviticus 15:19–30). This not only made her unable to participate in any religious service, but she was seen as "displeasing to God," and anyone and anything she touched (or anyone who touched what she had touched) was unclean. But Jesus not only healed the woman, he brought extraordinary attention to her.

It was obvious that Jesus wanted everyone to see that He thought more about the health, wholeness, and dignity of this woman than about what the religious rules and regulations said about her "uncleanness":

So he went with him. And a large crowd followed him and pressed in on him. Now there was a woman who had been suffering from hemorrhages for twelve years. She had endured much under many physicians, and had spent all that she had; and she was no better, but rather grew worse. She had heard about Jesus, and came up behind him in the crowd and touched his cloak, for she said, "If I but touch his clothes, I will be made well." Immediately her hemorrhage stopped; and she felt in her body that she was healed of her disease. Immediately aware that power had gone forth from him, Jesus turned about in the crowd and said, "Who touched my clothes?" And his disciples said to him, "You see the crowd pressing in on you; how can you say, 'Who touched me?' " He looked all around to see who had done it. But the woman, knowing what had happened to her, came in fear and trembling, fell down before him, and told him the whole truth. He said to her, "Daughter, your faith has made you well; go in peace, and be healed of your disease" (Mark 5:24–34; see also Matthew 9:10–26 and Luke 8:40–56).

What Made Jesus So Sensitive to Women?

When I think about how Jesus transcended the strict religious boundaries of Judaism, especially in His relationships with women, I cannot help but wonder why. Any psychiatrist, psychologist, or therapist of today worth her salt would begin examining a person's childhood and relationship with his or her parents for a clue or some insight into present-day behavior. But Jesus' birth occurred in a manner that defies the expected, traditional, religious, and ethical norms of that day. From his birth, a woman was doing the unexpected and accomplishing what seemed impossible to take care of Him.

Mary, Jesus' mother, risked her life, her engagement to Joseph, and her reputation to bring Him into this world. In Luke 1:28–35, we read of the totally unexpected. In Nazareth, a young girl, Mary, was engaged to Joseph. Everything in her life was going well until the angel Gabriel appeared to her:

> And the angel came in unto her, and said, Hail, thou that art highly favoured, the Lord is with thee: blessed art thou among women. And when she saw him, she was troubled at his saying, and cast in her mind what manner of salutation this should be. And the angel said unto her, Fear not, Mary: for thou hast found favour with God. And, behold, thou shalt conceive in thy womb, and bring forth a son, and shalt call his name Jesus. He shall be great, and shall be called the Son of the Highest: and the Lord God shall give unto him the throne of his father David: And he shall reign over the house of Jacob for ever; and of his kingdom there shall be no end. Then said Mary unto the angel, How shall this be, seeing I know not a man? [Isn't it funny that Mary is not shocked to see an angel; she's shocked because of the pregnancy part? I would be, too.] And the angel answered and said unto her, The Holy Ghost shall come upon thee, and the power of the Highest shall overshadow thee: therefore also that holy thing which shall be born of thee shall be called the Son of God (KJV).

There she was, a very young woman, living her life as other women her age, living the "expected" daily life of women in her culture and time. And without any warning, without any provocation or petitions to God on her part, Mary was chosen by God to bear the son of God, the Living Word.

Gabriel told her that she was the favored one of God. She is who God has chosen to fulfill God's will. Why can't this wait until *after* I am married to Joseph? Mary wondered. She was full of fear and apprehension; she knew what people would say. She knew the laws of her culture and religion. Worst of all, she knew that being found pregnant before marriage meant a sentence of death according to the Jewish Law.

The Jewish matrimonial procedure of betrothal consisted of two steps: a formal exchange of consent before witnesses (Malachi 2:14), and the subsequent taking of the bride to the groom's family home (Matthew 25:1–13). The first step was as legally binding as the second. The betrothal was usually entered into when the girl was between twelve and thirteen years old, and gave the young man rights over the girl. She was his wife, and any violation of his marital rights could be punished as adultery. Yet the wife continued to live at her own family home for about a year. Then the formal taking of the bride to the husband's family home occurred when he assumed her support. According to the Hebrew Law, if a bride was not a virgin, "then they shall bring the young woman out of the entrance of her father's house and the men of her town shall stone her to death" (Deuteronomy 22:21).

Mary feared for her life. The scandal would be unbearable, but she could survive scandal. However, the threat of death and the shame to her family were unthinkable! But God said it was possible!

Thousands of people have been given a vision of the utterly

unexpected and impossible to fulfill. Oftentimes only a few shared the vision or believed in the dream. Could it be possible that God does call women to preach? Could it be possible that God would come to us as men and women and need us to move outside of our comfort zones to do a new thing to change our church, our neighborhoods, and our world? Could God call us to change careers in midlife? Could God lead us to leave the company, its benefits, a guaranteed paycheck every other Friday, and begin using our forty hours a week doing something for which we have a passion?

Mary, after hearing the news that she was chosen to bear the child of God without the involvement of a man, asked, "How shall this be?" Gabriel answered, "The Holy Ghost shall come upon thee, and the power of the Highest shall overshadow thee; therefore also that holy thing which shall be born of thee shall be called the Son of God."

Women who feel called by God to preach, teach, or do something exceptionally new or extraordinary in their lives ask the same question as Mary: How can this be? How is it that I am to stand and speak, preach, or teach on behalf of God? Sometimes the question is born from a sense of unworthiness, our realization that God is holy and that we are humans with faults like everyone else. What makes us worthy? Like the prophet Isaiah, standing in the Temple before the presence of God, we, too, cry aloud, saying, "Woe is me! I am lost, for I am a [woman] of unclean lips, and I live among a people of unclean lips" (Isaiah 6:5). How shall this be? we ask. It shall be because of the Holy Spirit's anointing. "The Holy Ghost shall come upon thee and the power of the Highest will overshadow thee."

Sometimes it is not a feeling of unworthiness but rather a fear of success that keeps us from progressing in life. President Nelson Mandela said, "Our deepest fear is not that we are inadequate.

Our deepest fear is that we are powerful beyond measure. It is our light, not our darkness, that most frightens us." We try to control just about everything in our lives, but we cannot control the Spirit of God. We cannot tell God what to do, whom to use, and when or where to do His will. The Gospel of Jesus Christ is preached with such power that men and women, boys and girls come down the aisles of our churches every Sunday, accepting Jesus Christ as their Savior. God's spirit is powerful enough to seek and to save, powerful enough to wash us of all sins in the waters of baptism, but many still believe that God's Spirit is not powerful enough to use those same redeemed souls to proclaim the Good News that resides within their hearts.

When the possibilities of God are about to descend upon us, things that we do not understand happen. On the day of Pentecost, when the Holy Spirit fell upon everyone in the upper room, they began to proclaim God's praises in many tongues. The people said they must be drunk, but Peter stood and said:

> Men of Judea and all who live in Jerusalem, let this be known to you, and listen to what I say. Indeed, these are not drunk, as you suppose, for it is only nine o'clock in the morning. No, this is what was spoken through the prophet Joel: "In the last days it will be, God declares, that I will pour out my Spirit upon all flesh, and your sons and your daughters shall prophesy, and your young men shall see visions, and your old men shall dream dreams. Even upon my slaves, both men and women, in those days I will pour out my Spirit; and they shall prophesy" (Acts 2: 14–18).

When the power of the Most High overshadows you, that which is created inside is holy. Mary, overshadowed by the Spirit of God, conceives Jesus, the Christ. Women, anointed by the Spirit of God, conceive within their spirits the Good News that must be proclaimed. Women anointed by God's Spirit are free to be as creative as they possibly can, in order to bring some form of healing and wholeness to our world. If Mary had thought only about herself and her reputation, she may have refused to be the vessel for birthing Jesus into the world. Yet Mary believed that this child within her womb would save her people. She trusted that God would take care of her. Because God took care of Mary, Mary took care of the Christ Child.

God, the creator of the heavens and earth, chose to come to suffering humanity through the body of a woman! The One who created light out of darkness; the One who said "Let there be," and worlds leapt into existence; the One who, in the beginning, created man and woman from the dust of the earth—that One chose to come to us through a female vessel, a being not even thought to be fully human in her time, a person with no rights, oft abused, and even salable as property. The Living Word was to be delivered by a lowly maiden of the countryside!

One cannot help but empathize with the baffling emotions Mary must have been feeling at a time like this. And any woman called by God to an unexpected place in His plan feels this same fear, struggling against the sheer awe at the call of God. Mary dared not say no to the very emissary of God, so she reverently and, yes, timidly responded, "Behold the handmaid of the Lord: be it unto me according to thy word" (Luke 1:38 KJV).

Mary, filled with joy over being chosen by God, stood up to prophesy:

My soul doth magnify the Lord. And my spirit hath re-joiced in God my Saviour. For he hath regarded the low estate of his handmaiden: for, behold, from henceforth all generations shall call me blessed. For he that is mighty hath done to me great things; and holy is his name. And his mercy is on them that fear him from generation to generation. He hath shewed strength with his arm; he hath scattered the proud in the imagination of their hearts. He hath put down the mighty from their seats, and exalted them of low degree. He hath filled the hungry with good things; and the rich he hath sent empty away. He hath holpen his servant Israel, in remembrance of his mercy; as he spake to our fathers, to Abraham, and to his seed for ever (KJV).

If I may take a flight of imagination, I see Mary "opening the doors of the church," inviting all women and men to come and follow a God of possibilities. I can see them coming down through the ages, women and men who have accomplished things that others have called impossible. I see them coming from slavery— Sojourner Truth, Harriet Tubman, Gabriel Prosser. I see them coming from the arts—Marian Anderson, James Baldwin, Todd Duncan, Maya Angelou. I see them coming from the halls of education— Mary McLeod Bethune, George Washington Carver, Nannie Helen Burroughs. I see them coming from the halls of justice—Patricia Roberts Harris, Barbara Jordan, David Dinkins, Lawrence Douglas Wilder. I see them coming from the publications—Frederick Douglass, Ida B. Wells-Barnett, John H. Johnson. I see them coming from the athletic arena—Joe Louis, Althea Gibson, Jesse Owens, Tiger Woods, the Williams sisters. I see them coming from the church—Jarena Lee, Richard Allen, Martin Luther King Jr., Bishop Barbara Harris, Bishop Vashti Murphy McKenzie.

These are all lives that show the impossible possibilities of

God. They said yes when others wanted them t
something new and different when the rest of
ing the usual, expected routine. When pe.,
lives, their challenged beginnings, their race, their ¸
neighborhoods, everyone thought "impossible." A high-s.
dropout, a teenage mother, a prison record—impossible! How can
this be?

A teenage girl is pregnant. She is engaged to be married, but
the child is not her boyfriend's child, yet he marries her because
he loves her. He supports them both on his blue-collar income as a
carpenter. When she goes into labor, they are homeless. She gives
birth in a barn with animals as attendants and a stranger as mid-
wife. She gives birth to a son, whose life is threatened even from
birth because of his race and the possibility that he may one day
be a king and a deliverer of his people. In spite of all this, Mary
takes care of her son, Jesus, and he grows up to be a man who is
willing to break religious traditions to uplift the lives of all
women.

WOMEN IN JESUS' GENEALOGY

I believe Jesus was sensitive to the plight of women not only because of His mother, Mary, but also because of what His female
ancestors went through. You know what it's like when the family
gets together and someone starts telling stories about Aunt Bertie
and the secret circumstances of her son's birth. Maybe, when your
family gets together, there's always that one crazy cousin who
everyone prays did not receive the invitation. Every time he
shows up, some family secret is revealed, and it takes the whole
family tree years to bear fruit again.

Well, Jesus' family was no different. In Matthew 1:1–16, Jesus' genealogy is listed. But there is something unique about Jesus' genealogy—five women are included in the list. This is highly unusual. Women are not included in the genealogy of a man in the Jewish culture, but Jesus has five female ancestors listed, and they are not your run-of-the-mill apple-pie-baking aunties.

The first female ancestor's name is Tamar, in Matthew 1:3: "And Judah the father of Perez and Zerah by Tamar." Tamar's story is of soap opera proportions. (If you read the Bible, you will find enough sex, lies, and videotape to rival any Sidney Sheldon novel.) In Genesis, chapter 38, we are introduced to Tamar when she was given into marriage to Er, Judah's eldest son. This was an important family into which she married. Remember the patriarchs of Israel—Abraham, Isaac, and Jacob. Jacob had twelve sons who become the fathers of the twelve tribes of Israel, and Judah was the fourth of those sons. Judah had three sons—Er, Onan, and Shelah—and Tamar was Er's new wife. The Bible says that Er was wicked in the sight of the Lord and that the Lord slew him. I have no idea what Er did, but he pissed off the Almighty. So, since Tamar did not have the opportunity to bear sons for Er, Judah (the family patriarch) gave her to Onan, his next son. According to the Levite Law, it was Onan's responsibility to bear a son with Tamar in Er's name.

But that pairing didn't work out either (Onan met up with God's wrath, too). Judah, reluctant to pass Tamar on to his third and final son, Shelah, instead sent her back to live with her father until a later date. Tamar had her own ideas, though, and managed, eventually, to sleep with Judah himself (while she's masquerading as a prostitute) and get herself pregnant by him. As I said, all the makings of a soap opera. . . . (We will look at this story in much greater detail in chapter 6, "From Celibate to Celebrate.")

So, Auntie Tamar is in Jesus' genealogy. I'm sure knowing about her story influenced His attitude toward women who have had some sexual drama in their past.

The other four women in Jesus' genealogy were Rahab, a prostitute in Jericho who helped the Israelite spies escape to safety (Joshua 2:1–24); Ruth, who manipulated a nighttime situation with a wealthy man and became the grandmother of King David (Ruth); Bathsheba, who had an adulterous affair with King David, resulting in the murder of her husband (II Samuel 11:3–5); and Mary, his mother. All five of these women had some sexual indiscretion in their lives. These women have very dark pasts including incest, prostitution, unwed motherhood, questionable virginity at marriage, adultery, and accomplice to murder. But if it were not for them, there would be no Jesus. Our Savior came through their bloodline. So it's no wonder Jesus was sensitive to the woman caught in the act of adultery. And we should not be surprised that he was comfortable eating and drinking with prostitutes and sinners. He could be compassionate to the widow of Nain, whose son died, because he knew his own mother would soon have to experience the death of a son. He knew the shame and guilt the Samaritan woman at the well experienced every day she came to draw water and had to endure the stares and whispers of the other women who knew that she was living with a man who was not her husband—and there had been five others before him.

Jesus understands women. Jesus listens to women and Jesus loves women.

It excites me every time I think about the women who followed Jesus and the disciples: Mary Magdalene, Susanna, and Joanna. What in the world could it have been like to be in Jesus' entourage? Sitting around in the evening when dinner is over, usually the men and the women separate into different parts of the house, but now Jesus invites the sisters to stay near and share their thoughts and experiences. Jesus lets them know that the Kingdom of God has a place for them, too.

It was no accident but Divine Will that, just as Jesus took care of the sisters when He was alive, the sisters took care of Jesus while He was dying. Can't you imagine the agony and horror of watching a brother like Jesus being falsely accused, tried by a kangaroo court, beaten all night long. There He stood—alone, betrayed by Judas, denied by Peter. But as He bore a wooden cross on His shoulders up Golgotha's hill, it was the women and John who walked with Him.

This crucifixion scene reminds me of the movie *Steel Magnolias*. M'Lynn's daughter Shelby has died. Standing by the grave with her SisterFriends, M'Lynn shares the last moments of Shelby's life. She speaks in whispered tones saying how blessed she felt for being there when that little life came into the world and being there when she left. "It's funny, men are supposed to be made of steel or something, but the men left, it was just me and Shelby. Women are like steel magnolias." Yes, women are strong, we can endure the hardships and pains of life and live on to proclaim the Good News of Easter morning—Jesus lives!

What is your favorite story in the Bible about Jesus? Why?

_____

_____

_____

_____

_____

If Jesus were walking the earth today as an African American minister, what kind of man would He be? As a religious leader, what issues would He address and how?

_____

_____

_____

_____

_____

List men alive today whom you feel treat women with the respect and honor as Jesus did in His time and culture. These can be public figures or personal acquaintances.

_____

_____

_____

_____

If you were one of the women who followed Jesus like Mary Magdalene, Joanna, or Susanna, about what would you talk with Jesus? What do you think it would be like to be Jesus' confidante and friend?

_____

_____

_____

_____

CHAPTER FOUR

Reclaiming Our Bodies—From the Auction Block, to the Altar, and Beyond

African American women's history in this country goes back to the auction block. Standing there, our bodies stripped naked, in full view of everyone, we were put on display and seen as objects. We were property. We had no rights to our own bodies, and white traders were allowed to touch and explore us, looking for some blemish that would reduce our value, as if we were cattle for sale.

Dr. Gail E. Wyatt, author of *Stolen Women: Reclaiming Our Sexuality, Taking Back Our Lives*, says, "What happened on that auction block centuries ago is still unfinished business for African American women today. In a society increasingly obsessed with sex, too many people—white and black—still hold this dangerous view: that black women must either ignore their sexuality altogether or be perpetually sexually available."

Slave women had no rights to their own bodies. At any time a white man could force himself upon a slave woman without any repercussions. She was his property, and he could do as he pleased with her. A girl's first sexual experience was likely to be rape; therefore, virginity was not expected of black women. Black women had to submit to any white man who made sexual demands on them; otherwise, they would be beaten or their family would be punished. Black women as slaves had to use sex to keep their babies with them and to keep their men alive. The result of sustaining such experiences is the development of a negative image of one's body. It was the naked bodies of slave women that our collective memory has internalized. To see the nakedness of our foremothers is to remember the horror, pain, and shame of slavery. For many women today, there are still shame and negative feelings associated with being naked. Some women will not let their partners see them undress. Some women will only have sex in the dark so their bodies will not be seen. Unfortunately, many women have chosen simply to cover up their bodies, believing that any clothing that is revealing is what "bad girls" wear.

Marilyn Hughes Gaston, M.D., and Gayle K. Porter, Psy.D., in their book *Prime Time: The African American Woman's Complete Guide to Midlife Health and Wellness*, state, "Our ability as Black women to view our sexuality in a healthy manner, as an important part of our body, mind, and spirit, has been seriously compromised by racism, culture, ageism, homophobia, and religion." From the post–Civil War days up to the early sixties the South was notorious for lynching blacks. The majority of the victims were men, but some women were hanged, too. Billie Holliday sang about it, saying, "Southern trees bear strange fruit." This terrorizing image of black people was emblazoned upon the mind and memory of every kidnapped child of Africa. If we did not witness the lynching, our parents or grandparents did. Somewhere among our ancestors, someone—with our eyes, our lips, our ears, our faces—stood as an eyewitness to white America's inhumanity to our bodies and souls.

Dr. Cornel West, in his book *Race Matters*, says in the chapter titled "On Black Sexuality," "This white dehumanizing endeavor has left its toll in the psychic scars and personal wounds now inscribed in the souls of black folk. These scars and wounds are clearly etched on the canvas of black sexuality."

As black people we have 254 years of slavery, Jim Crow, and lynching, with the sole purpose of devaluing our people. Thanks be to God for people and places in our culture and community where we were loved and encouraged to love ourselves. We should give thanks every day for HBCUs (Historically Black Colleges and Universities), black fraternities and sororities, the Black church, black barbershops and beauty salons, and every person, place, or thing that affirmed black people as beautiful, intelligent people with a capacity to survive slavery and succeed at anything we put our hands to. We should thank God daily for our wise elders who lived through slavery and knew how important it was to tell a child, "Baby, you is beautiful."

We must also reclaim our bodies and ourselves from the stereotypes people have used to label us. Not only were African Americans seen and treated as objects and their bodies abused as slaves, but once someone labels you a particular thing, it takes years for others to see you as anything different. It is important for women to define themselves, not based solely upon what they look like, but based on who they really are as a collective and unique gender, and also as individual personalities.

The evil that one people is able to commit against another people is inconceivable. Further, it is even more amazing to see how these acts of evil become a part of our soulful heritage and a memorial in our mind. As a young girl, I read *The Diary of Anne Frank*; shortly thereafter, I saw a documentary about the Nazi concentration camp of Auschwitz. I was horrified by what I saw in this documentary—the physical and psychological afflictions endured by the Jews. Of all their horrors, the one that stayed with my subconscious was the labeling of the prisoners. Jews wore a yellow patch in the shape of a Star of David; homosexuals wore an inverted, pink triangle—which they have now transformed into a symbol of gay pride. I don't know when it happened, but somewhere between undergraduate school and seminary, I refused to wear a name badge. As a minister, I am always attending conferences, church seminars, and women's social groups, where it is standard procedure to register, receive your information packet, and put on a name badge. I could not and will not do it. A resistance is within me. I refuse to have someone identify me by a 3×3 card pinned on my jacket, Velcroed to my dress, or hung around my neck. If you want to know who I am, ask me.

In Spike Lee's movie *Bamboozled*, there is a scene in which Manray and Womack are preparing to apply burned cork to their skin in order to perform in blackface. The first time they did it with some hesitation, but they were able to perform because the show was popular and they were "getting pa-zaid." But as time progressed, it became evident that this process of applying blackface was not only changing the complexion of their skin, but also darkening their spirits.

In many black music videos, women are portrayed in sexually explicit, demeaning ways—they are purely sex objects. Similar to exotic dancers at what are called "booty clubs," these sisters are objectified. They dance, gyrate their bodies, and expose the most private and intimate areas of themselves in order to sexually entertain, arouse, and excite men for money. These women are not seen as "my sisters in Christ" or "children of God" at these clubs— they are sex objects. They are instruments for men's sexual desires. This industry succeeds on the knowledge that men will pay a lot of money for a three- to five-minute lap dance. The men are not allowed to touch the women (right!) or engage in any sexual activity in the club. Sisters need to reclaim their bodies.

When I was pastoring First Congregational United Church of Christ in Atlanta, Georgia, there was a popular downtown strip club behind my church. Our two buildings were separated by the church's very large parking lot. The owner of the club was a relative of one of the families of the church. We met at his aunt's funeral and became friends. I could not believe that this "nice" brother owned and operated a booty club. He had another traditional business in medical supplies, but he said, "I make more money with my clubs." I asked him if the women who worked for him were taken care of. He said that they had health insurance and that the bouncers made sure they were not treated inappropriately. I told him that if any of the sisters needed counseling or had a problem, I was available to help. No one ever called.

I've asked various men who I know frequent these clubs, "You're married, why do you go to the club?" They give various reasons, but my favorite one is, "Most of these girls are college students and need the money to pay their tuition." I guess he never thought of going to the bursar's office or the financial-aid office and making a donation.

Dancing and the Black Church

Dancing has been just as taboo as sex in the realm of the church. The only dancing that is allowed is the *holy* dance, which is observed when a person is under the influence of the Holy Spirit and dances in praise of God, or liturgical dance, where dancing is done as an interpretation of sacred music in worship. Throughout the years there has been great concern about the morals of people who dance. Parents of every generation have tried to discourage young people from doing certain *nasty* dances. Dances such as the dirty dog, da Butt, dirty dancing, and the Freak have all been frowned upon by various generations. The major fear is that young people will become sexually active because of these dances. However, dancing is a healthy outlet for those raging hormones. When kids party together with their friends, they are together in a community with others, not isolated and alone somewhere.

At dances and parties we developed many of our social skills with the opposite sex. There was the excitement of what to wear to a party, who was going to be there, whether someone would ask you for your phone number, and if you would be asked to dance. These were all great emotional concerns, the outcome of which was dependent not just on your personality but on your body as well.

When I was in junior high and high school, I remember how important it was to look good when going to a party or dance. My girlfriend and I would go to one store to get the pants, another store to get a top, another store for the shoes, and yet another store for the jewelry. At the end of the day I had my elephant-leg or bell-bottom pants; a popcorn, zip-up-the-front bodysuit that snapped at the crotch; my platform shoes; and my dolphin-kissing, gold-painted hoop earrings. I had to look good so someone would ask me to dance. The parties were usually held at my sister's class-mate's house. There were black lights (that were really purple), posters, punch, and snacks. The black lights made our afros look as if they had been dusted with lint.

We all brought our 45s, our names painted on their labels with fingernail polish. The Delfonics, Blue Magic, or the Chi-Lites would begin singing, and we began slow dragging, or dancing on a dime as some would call it. If you were lucky, someone you were attracted to would ask you to dance, and afterward, you'd go to the bathroom with your girlfriends and squeal about how good it felt to dance with Maurice, Keith, Peter, or Patrick. It was always so dark at these house parties. After dancing with the same guy all night, you were in love. When the host called out, "Last dance!" everyone grabbed that special someone and slowly moved to the Dells' "Stay in My Corner." Everyone slowly climbed up the steps from the basement into the light of the kitchen, and suddenly you realized that Prince Charming had turned into a frog! He'd ask for your phone number, and you'd give him the number of Coastline Cab Company.

For many, dancing at house parties was our introduction to sharing our sexual feelings and navigating the waters of these emotions. We began to realize the impact and influence our bodies had on the opposite sex. But we did not see our bodies or dancing as anything sinful or wrong. But the next morning, after having danced away Saturday night, we would come to church and hear words of condemnation about the wiles of the devil and the sins that occur when we "shake that thang."

Dance is a wonderful and central part of any celebration for Africans in America, as well as all African people. In 1992, the United Church of Christ Board for World Ministries sent several college students and adults to West Africa. One of the most joyous memories for me is the dancing. In the village of Ho, in the Volta region of Ghana, we stayed with the people in a compound. We rose early in the morning to gather for prayer. Some of us worked in the fields, helping to plant crops before the rainy season; others helped in building their church. At noon we came in to eat and rest, for it was too hot to be outside working. In the evening, after dinner, some people would come from a nearby village and bring their drums, and we would dance for two or three hours. The black students and adults from the United States did the electric slide to the drumming, and one of the Ghanaians said, "Oh, we thank our American brothers and sisters for their gift of this wonderful dance." They thought we'd prepared this choreographed dance for them. They did not know that we had never danced together as a group before that evening. But that is what dance is— a gift. Dance is basic for all celebrations and rituals for Africans.

We all have enjoyed the talents and dancing genius of Bill Bojangles Robinson, Katherine Dunham, Josephine Baker, Ben Vereen, the Dance Theater of Harlem, Gregory Hines, Alvin Ailey, Savion Glover, and thousands of others. It is not the dance that destroys one's life, it is the interpretation and limitations that are projected upon the dance. Dancing is an expression and celebration of life for black people.

As a pastor, I have always found it refreshing to attend a Saturday-night celebration at the home of a church member and see people of every age dancing and having a good time. Seeing my church members celebrating added a new dimension to them for me on Sunday morning. Why do we try to separate ourselves in such a way? There is nothing different about the Susan who does the electric slide on Saturday and the Susan who celebrates Holy Communion on Sunday. It was the wisest man who ever lived, King Solomon, who put it so succinctly: "To every thing there is a season, and a time to every purpose under the heaven . . . a time to mourn, and a time to dance" (Ecclesiastes 3:1, 4 KJV).

The uniqueness of line dancing or group dancing is that you don't need a partner. You are able to dance in community with others. There is no rejection, no challenge to your self-esteem if no special someone asks you to dance—you don't need a partner. This frees you up to go on and do "your thang." You can be creative with your body without being concerned about what your partner thinks. You are free to express your sensuality in a way that is okay. You don't need anyone to affirm you by asking you to dance, you affirm yourself; and while you are dancing, you express an aspect of your sexuality in a celebratory way.

Children possess a great freedom in dance. Think about your family get-togethers and the little two-year-old baby girl who begins to move to the beat of music playing. The adult women laugh and say, "Go on, baby girl, do your thang!" We encourage children to enjoy this form of self-expression. We get joy out of seeing them so freely celebrate their bodies. Children are fully integrated with body, spirit, and soul. We all were fully integrated at one time, but somewhere in our lives we internalized the opinions of others. Somewhere in our lives we were told not to "shake your big behind like that." Someone spoke a negative word to us about our bodies, and we began to equate dancing with something negative, and to view our bodies, the instruments of dance, as sinful. We took these words of doubt, shame, and discouragement, and we internalized them and nurtured them. Later when we'd start to feel good about ourselves, we'd trot out these doubts and hang them around our necks, or bind them around our wrist and wear them like the shackles they'd become. We became comfortable with our doubts. We update them from time to time like a new variation to an ancient sacred theme, but the original tune of discouragement can always be recognized. We wear these negative feelings like a charm bracelet, each year adding something new. But we were born in total innocent freedom, and somewhere in our lives something was said or done that made us begin to diminish ourselves in some way. But the good news is that she that the Son has made free, is free indeed!

SAYING "I DO" WHEN YOU DON'T

Another area where some women need to reclaim their bodies is in the marriage relationship. Throughout the years we have tried to bring dignity back to our nakedness. We have happily bought into the ideal that by wearing white and becoming a man's bride, we could stand virginal at the altar and be redeemed. To counter the images of promiscuity prevalent today, some black women adopt very restrictive sexual practices as single women and as married women. Some women feel that marriage will redeem their bodies, then, after getting married, they realize that this is not the answer.

A greater number of women than men try to hold to the practice of not enjoying sexual intimacies until after marriage. Because of this, we find that some women, whose religious affiliation teaches no sex outside of marriage, are consumed with finding a husband. Again, there still exists a double moral standard for men and women regarding sexual intimacies before marriage. Women are expected to remain abstinent; men, on the other hand, are expected to be men. So good Christian women are under duress trying to maintain this good-girl image and to hurry up and get married to satisfy their natural sexual desires.

So for these women, every man who asks them out on a date is automatically sized up as a potential mate. After dating for a period of time, many women are ready for him to pop the question—will you marry me?

This expectation is greater for women who have been sexually intimate with their men. They have shared a special part of themselves that, from childhood, they've been taught should only be shared in the marriage bed. So the pressure is on to get married. It is almost like a video game in which one must master a certain level before the game will give you access to the next level. We do play games with relationships, whether consciously or unconsciously. Once a sister has been asked out on a date, the game of courtship is afoot. Level one of the game is getting along with each other, learning about each other's likes, dislikes, families, occupations, hobbies, income. We have ways of finding out a brother's income. Level one can last anywhere from one week to two months. Level two is when the sister invites him to meet her girlfriends or to some family event like a Sunday dinner, a reunion, a cousin's wedding, etc. This gives her an opportunity to see how he interacts with her people, and her people get an opportunity to size him up and report back to her. "Yeah girl, I think this is the one," the women may say.

Level three is when she wants him to come to church and/or church-sponsored functions on her arm. Level three is so distinctive, you can recognize it immediately. A woman who usually comes to church alone and sits with her friends all of a sudden enters the sanctuary with an unknown soldier (a brother-in-training for husband material) on her arm, and she sits in a different place. She fusses over him as if he's never been to church before. She turns to the morning hymn for him, and they share the same hymnbook. She provides him with an offering envelope. She speaks to folks she's never spoken to in order to introduce her friend. Oh yes, and when it is time for altar prayer, she takes him by the hand, and they go to the altar and pray together. He has no idea that this is a rehearsal for him to get used to the idea of standing at the church altar with her, in front of all her friends and family. Don't get mad at me, you know it's the truth!

I'm not saying that women are consciously manipulating men to marry them, for we all know that a black man doesn't do anything he doesn't want to do (unless we get a little something from Miss Rudolph, the root worker—just kidding, saints!). But by now, they are known as a couple. At any function, if some other woman is seen talking to her man, she suddenly has a need to ask him a question or fall into a simulated, fused version of This Is My Man and Back Off! I preached at a church in Maryland a few weeks ago; after the service, the pastor invited me to his daughter's engagement party. Everyone in attendance had been at the worship services that morning. Some were preparing the food, some were in one room talking, and some of us were in the TV room looking at the NBA playoffs. As I was talking with a brother about the skilled Allen Iverson, a young sister almost sat in my lap to get between me and her man. She said, "Honey, can I get you some dessert?" He replied, "No, I'm not eating any dessert today, got to get back in the gym." He then continued to talk to me around her body about basketball; it was very awkward, but she was not moving. Later, she did leave, but when she returned I could tell she was miffed because her man was eating dessert.

This is the level in the game of courtship where it gets emotionally taxing for both people. She's been acting like his wife, talking like his wife, doing things with and for him like his wife, but she's *not* his wife. She's frustrated and begins to let him know it. At this point, the brother has to survive the holiday hurdles. You know the holiday hurdles—that period of time between Thanksgiving and Valentine's Day that a man has to survive without getting engaged. If a man and woman have dated through all three levels, then they are faced with the holiday hurdles. Each player has a different task to accomplish in order to master this level. The man must celebrate Thanksgiving, Christmas, New Year's Eve, New Year's Day, Kwanzaa, her birthday (if it falls between November and February), and Valentine's Day with his girlfriend without asking her to marry him.

The woman's objective in the holiday hurdles is to use any possible method or charm to get him to propose marriage to her between November and February. If his birthday falls during this period, she has to pull out all the stops and let him know how wonderful his life would be if he were married to her. By this time, all her girlfriends, coworkers, and family members have been listening to her extol this brother's worth; they see the relationship through her eyes, so everyone expects an engagement. Oftentimes, everyone *except* the man expects it. Male and female perspectives on the things of life are very different (see chapter 6, "From Celibate to Celebrate").

One Sunday after service, a church member pulled me aside to ask if he could come to me for counseling. I agreed and we made an appointment for that Wednesday. Charles is an attractive thirty-four-year-old, single black man who has been dating another member of the church for eight months. In the session he told me, "Dr. Newman, Sharon is pressuring me into getting married, and I'm just not ready for that. When we started dating eight months ago, she was my first real girlfriend in three years, and I'm used to being by myself and having my time to myself. I love her, but she demands so much of me." I asked him if he'd shared his feelings with Sharon and he said, "Yes, I've told her and she says she understands, but she doesn't change any of her behavior; she still does everything the same."

Most of the church members have noticed that they come to church together on Sundays and Wednesday nights. Instead of sitting with the other deacons-in-training, Charles has been sitting with Sharon during worship. They go to the altar together for prayer. They sponsor potluck dinners at his or her home for their friends. They appear to be a happy Christian couple, but Charles was not totally happy. I asked him if he'd like for me to counsel with him and Sharon, but he declined and said he'd talk with her again. A few months later, Charles became an ordained deacon; and two weeks after that, Sharon announced their engagement. Sharon was ecstatic; Charles just smiled.

In conversations with some of the single women at the church, Sharon would boast about her relationship with Charles. They were sexually abstinent, waiting to share themselves with each other on their wedding night. She would not even allow Charles to French-kiss her. The day after Charles proposed to her, Sharon set up a website with all the information about their wedding plans. She'd been planning this wedding for a while.

This would all be so romantic and wonderful if both partners felt the same throughout the courtship. But even now when I see Charles and Sharon, she's still just as ecstatic about the approaching nuptials, and Charles is still just smiling. I wonder how long he'll be smiling after the wedding.

It is important to marry for life-nurturing, healthy, and loving reasons. Don't marry because you feel pressure of any kind. Please do not marry because you're withholding sexual intimacy from your life until marriage. Marriage is a relationship that a couple enters into for mutual enjoyment; it marks the beginning of a shared lifetime. It is important that both people have the same desire to share their lives and agree to talk about each other's expectations in love and respect. You may not always agree with what the other desires, but it is important to speak honestly about your wants and mutually agree upon the best way to move forward in the spirit of love to achieve them together.

Another aspect of marriage that we need to look at is the fact that a wedding ceremony does not come with a guarantee of great sex. Some women can't wait to get married, so they can freely give themselves to their husbands because "the [marriage] bed [is] undefiled" (Hebrews 13:4). Well, not only is the marriage bed undefiled, for some it is unsatisfactory as well.

Many single women tend to believe that once a woman is married, everything will be all right. She has her man, and the sex is free-flowing and wonderful. *Not!* When relationships are new, there is passion and magic. Each and every word your beloved utters is precious, every act of kindness is a gift, and every gift is a treasure. But after you're married and the glow and excitement of the courtship and wedding have worn off, after the honey in the honeymoon has dried up, the realities of married life set in. It's not easy to keep passion in the bedroom 365/24/7 with a person with whom you pay bills, raise children, and argue about the toilet seat being left up. But it *can* be done.

Once the magic wears off, then the work in a relationship begins. Sisters work all day, come home and prepare dinner, help the kids complete their homework, and get the kids washed up and in bed. Usually there is something from the office that she needs to review for tomorrow's meeting, or research and reading that she needs to do for that class she's taking at the university. After all this, it's time to become this sex goddess who looks like Janet Jackson, Jennifer Lopez, or all three of Destiny's Children, all rolled up into one woman, 'cause you know fantasy is a big part of a brother's libido.

Well, the truth is that women want a sex god in the bedroom, too. They fantasize about Morris Chestnut, Taye Diggs, Denzel Washington, Maxwell and Tyson Beckford, all rolled up into one, too. But the reality is that it's just you and your spouse together. The key is to find ways to please each other before you get to the bedroom. I always believe in doing little loving things all day long that will explode into a wonderful session of lovemaking later that night.

Start off by making a date with your husband. Plan it for a Friday night when the kids can have a sleepover with friends or a relative. That Friday morning, before he leaves for work, put a love note in his briefcase, or send him an erotic e-mail during the day. It is always good for the man to send flowers to his lady as a midday preview of the evening's romance as well. You can plan to go out for dinner, so no one has to do the cooking. All during dinner you can act in loving and alluring ways by feeding each other and holding hands (something we forget to do after marriage). And there is nothing like the smile on your man's face when you slip off your shoe and stroke his leg with your foot.

There are so many options one has between dinner and the act of lovemaking. Depending on the area where you live, you could go for a drive by the water, take a walk in a nice romantic area, or go home and slow dance to your favorite love songs. Whatever you do, remember that lovemaking begins before the bed, that is, if you make it to the bedroom. It is often more exciting to make love in other places in the home rather than your usual place—try it, you might surprise yourself. Remember, you are two consenting adults; if your partner agrees with whatever you want to do, go for it!

Communication is a lost art. Some folks just don't want to talk about sex, then they complain about not being sexually fulfilled. No one can read your mind and know what feels good to you; you've got to tell them.

Recently I was counseling a couple who were about to get married. Mark and Katrina were both very attractive people in their late twenties. He was from Wisconsin and she was from California. They met at a mutual friend's party and hit it off. They dated for a year, then got engaged and moved in together three months before the wedding. As a part of premarital counseling I always devote an entire session to the sexual and intimate aspects of the couple's relationship.

I asked them, "How is your sex life?" Mark answered, "It's great, Katrina is a good lover." Katrina answered in a melancholy voice, "It's all right." Then Mark, as if Katrina's response gave him permission to be honest, said, "Well, the truth is, I like it, but sometimes I feel that she would rather be painting her nails or watching television." Katrina responded, "Sometimes I would." At this point, I knew this was an area that needed some help. We talked further and it was revealed that Mark rushes through lovemaking without much foreplay, and that he has an orgasm and is finished before Katrina gets warmed up. This is a common experience for many women. Some women never tell their lovers, "Wait! I'm not finished!"

If your lover really cares about sex being as fulfilling and enjoyable to you as it is for him, then he will be more than willing to talk about how to improve upon the time spent and ways to approach sex differently. There are therapists who specialize in counseling and coaching individuals and couples with sexual dysfunctions or couples who simply need some help in having a more complete sexual relationship. (See the "Resources" section.)

Dr. June Dobbs-Butts, a sexual therapist and educator in

Atlanta, Georgia, suggests one refreshing technique for couples. Dr. Butts tells the man and woman to take turns initiating the lovemaking session: the man gets the odd-numbered days and the woman the even-numbered days. On these days, if one of them wants to spend time with the other, enjoying the pleasures of their bodies, then he or she is to invite the partner to the bed. The ground rules are as follows: 1) no touching or direct stimulation of the genital area, 2) only the day's initiator can explore, kiss, and touch the other partner, 3) the couple may massage each other, hold each other, and kiss, but may do nothing to directly bring each other to orgasm. The goal of this exercise is for a couple to spend time getting to know each other's body and figuring out what touches can arouse and please the partner besides direct stimulation of the genital area and penetration. Dr. Butts suggests that couples do this for a week, and when they come back for counseling, they can discuss what happened and whether it made a difference.

Well, I suggested this touching session to Mark and Katrina. After a week of this exercise, when they came into my office, they were holding hands and sitting close together on the sofa. This was very different from the earlier session, when they'd sat separately on the sofa, not touching at all. They said that they enjoyed the exercise and discovered things that aroused them that they never knew about before. Katrina liked the privilege of initiating the touching session.

A lot of women were raised to feel that they are not supposed to enjoy sex, that sex is only for a man's enjoyment. This is not true. Women do enjoy sex as much as men do, and it is okay for a woman to be the initiator and aggressor in sexual relations. A lot of men would really be turned on if their lovers initiated the lovemaking. Tell your lover what you like, how you like it, and for how long. Don't be shy about expressing your erotic nature; it is one of the most liberating experiences in life. There are women who have had children but have never had an orgasm. Take time to get to know your own body and find out what arouses you; then tell your beloved. If you need a little help, go see a sex therapist. For some it may be a little embarrassing at first, but so was your first Pap smear; look at it like this, with a little help and patience, and you will discover the joy and ecstasy of orgasm.

RECLAMATION FROM THE CULTURE

The Psalmist wrote, "[We are] fearfully and wonderfully made" (Psalm 139). God made us in God's image and said it is good, so who are we to deny our beauty? We need to reclaim our bodies from what the fashion world holds up as the standard of beauty. A great number of women are critical about some aspect of their bodies without any help from advertisers. They already stand in front of the mirror and look at their flabby arms, their thunder thighs, their breasts that need to be held in a blouse with a safety pin or breasts that qualify their owners for membership in the Itty Bitty Titty Committee. Some women have petite feet and others have Barney Rubble feet. No matter what level of self-esteem women have about their bodies, when the advertisers finish unleashing their targeted ads, many women receive the intended messages loud and clear: "You are not good enough . . . and you can fix yourself only if you buy our product." There are many women who are trying to reimage their bodies to look like the front cover of a fashion magazine. The beauty icon of the fashion industry is a woman whose dress size is between a one and a six. I ain't got nothing on my body that's a size six.

Our entire culture is obsessed with weight loss, not for health reasons but for aesthetics. Women are more adversely affected by size and weight than men. A girlfriend told me about responding to a personal ad in the paper (really, it wasn't me) in which a man described himself as having an athletic build; when he showed up she realized that he was not referring to football but to sumo wrestling. Women, on the other hand, are hardly ever described as having an athletic build. We are called fat, thick, chubby, or just big. I've learned to accept the body I'm in, until I can exercise it to a healthier body. I tell people, "I'm in shape . . . round is a shape." For years women like me have delayed enjoying ourselves and our lives because we were waiting to be a size six, or a size ten, or whatever size we thought would bring us nirvana. There are three areas of concern for most men when it comes to their body—baldness, impotence, and a big gut (the latter is not as important as the first two). Advertisers have a field day with men on products like Rogaine and Viagra. For many black men, hair is not an issue; brothers are going with the Isaac Hayes/Michael Jordan look—bold, black, and bald. Women, on the other hand, have hundreds of self-improvement products.

I have personally sacrificed my body to the weight-loss industry for the last forty years, and I have lost and gained the same sixty pounds in each millennium. I've been on the grapefruit diet, cabbage soup diet, high protein diet, low carbohydrate diet, and a vegetarian diet. I've done Scarsdale, Atkins, the Zone, Sugar Busters, Jenny Craig, Optifast, Slimfast, and Metabolife. I've had a gastric bubble in my belly and staples in my stomach. I've been a member of Weight Watchers six times since I was twelve years old. I have now been put out of Weight Watchers and cannot join anywhere in the world. I'm sure if they put my name in the computer, Mace would spray out.

In the 1980s I joined the organization for the sixth time, trying once again to lose weight. I was still trying to look like the women in *Essence* and *Ebony*. At that time you could join Weight Watchers if you were at least ten pounds over your goal weight. I weighed in at 235 pounds. I got all my materials and eating guidelines and went home, ready to lose five pounds by the next week. The week passed, and I wanted to lose so bad that I hardly ate anything. I went to my meeting and stood on the scale, and this wiry woman maneuvered the weights across the bar, fussing with the one-hundred-pound marker, knowing that I ain't weighed in the one hundreds since I learned my times tables.

She finally looked in my book, positioned the markers at 235 pounds, then flicked the marker slightly to the right: 234¼ pounds. I couldn't believe it! I had lived off steamed air and dehydrated water for seven days and I lost only three-quarters of a pound! I was livid when I went into the meeting. Members were going around testifying about how much they'd lost or gained. Some received applause for losses and others got sympathetic nods and words of encouragement for gains. I was still livid. Then this six-foot, blond woman, an airline attendant who could have lost ten pounds simply by removing her lipstick and hair spray, stood up and whined, "I've gained a half pound." Well, I let out a whoop and applauded, saying, "Yes, yes!" The class leader scolded me, "Susan!" I said, "Well, look at her, she's got to run around in the shower to get wet." My attitude was not acceptable, and I had to leave the meeting. I have since made a "searching and fearless inventory of myself" and have realized that expressing a bad attitude toward another does not improve my lot. But I still want to be in the *Jet* magazine centerfold; I'd wear a two-piece ensemble—a swimsuit and a trench coat.

One day I had an "aha moment" and realized that I cannot be

anyone else but me. Being who I am is very much a part of being in my body. I may not be Halle Berry, but I'm hallelujah to a couple of brothers. I have to be excited about the skin I'm in. If we don't think our bodies are beautiful, we shouldn't expect anyone else to see them as beautiful. Think about what some women sacrifice on the altar of vanity in order to have acceptable bodies. Some have had tummy tucks, liposuction, breast implants, body wraps, and so forth.

As in all things of Spirit, when you learn to be at peace with some aspect of yourself, then you've arrived. Eleanor Roosevelt once said, and I paraphrase, "It is not important by what name people call you, but rather, to what name you answer." There will always be outside critical voices ready to announce to the world who you are and how you and your body image have fallen short of some standard or expectation. When this happens, just proclaim, "Get your traditions off my body." Refuse to wear the garments of ancient opinions. Throw off the false mantle and adorn yourself with the vestments of your true identity.

Speaking of garments, we need to reclaim our bodies from the pressure to buy and wear everything this culture says is *in*. It may be *in* for some, but it may be *out* for you. A lot of women don't think before they purchase an outfit. They see it on a mannequin and decide it will look just as good on them. My first rule is: If it's made of spandex, you should put it down and walk away quietly. Just because it comes in your size does not mean you should buy it. What we put on should enhance our natural beauty and sensuality, not be all there is to our beauty. The same thing applies to hair and makeup. Television commercials and magazine ads will entice you to believe that blond, red, or maroon hair will look good on you. Take a moment and think about this before you go and permanently dye your hair. Try a wig on first to see how you look—the mirror does not lie, so don't lie to yourself. Everything is not for every*body*. Don't misunderstand me, I'm all for women doing what they can to enhance their natural beauty. A dear friend and cosmetologist, Montagus Portee, used to say "There's enough powder and paint to make you the woman you ain't." There's no excuse for any woman not to look her best. You don't have to wear all of the makeup on your bathroom counter. But there is nothing like going to a salon and getting the works—hair, makeup, manicure, pedicure, a massage! Be prepared to spend at least $100 for just two of these experiences, but I think you're worth it. Save up for this, as you would do for a concert. When I first saw RuPaul, I knew I could do better with what God gave me.

RECLAIMING OUR BODIES FROM THE CHURCH

The Catholic Church is opposed to any form of contraception except by natural means, of *self*-control. The Catholic Church is opposed to birth control pills, condoms, IUDs, foams, jellies, sterilization, coitus interruptus—or any other means used to prevent conception from resulting from this act—because "such means profane the marital embrace and dishonor the marriage contract."

The Catholic Church believes that the conception of children is the ultimate purpose for which God created sexuality. Sexual union is a gift from God to the married, but by practicing contraception, married couples are accepting the pleasure God built into the act and yet denying Him its purpose, which is new people. Those who have a true and serious need to space or limit the number of their children are instructed to rely upon natural family planning based on periodic abstinence.

Well, this just doesn't sit well with me. The Catholic Church cannot dictate to me what I can and cannot do with my body. The day I turn on Headline News and discover the story of the day is "The Pope's period is late! Details at eleven!" is the day I will be glad to sit down and discuss birth control with him. Then I will feel as if I am getting advice from someone who knows what he's talking about. I will be talking to someone who understands the anguish a woman goes through when she misses her period. I will then be speaking with someone who knows the anxiety of wondering, Am I pregnant? But until then, the Pope and the members of the Catholic Church's Bishop's Council and any other man can express their opinions about my ovaries, fallopian tubes, and womb, but I don't have to listen. I have that kind of conversation with my SisterFriends and my God.

In reclaiming our bodies from the dictums of the church, women of spirit must insist on the support and respect of religious leaders to help them achieve the following:

- access to comprehensive, age-appropriate information about sexuality and reproduction
- good, affordable health care to ensure a safe pregnancy and delivery
- access to health services to help the infertile achieve pregnancy
- counseling and resources to help a woman plan when it is in her best interest to conceive a child and how many she wants to conceive
- access to the full range of contraceptive services and appropriate information about reproduction
- access to health care that is safe and effective

Our body was our only possession when we came into this world, and when we go, we will leave it behind. But until then, let's take the best care of ourselves that we can. Let us begin today to love ourselves a little more. Talk to your body, affirm it, nourish it, exercise it, bathe it, moisturize it, perfume it; be gentle with yourself and do not allow anyone else to do any harm to it. Your body is a temporary temple for your journey on this earth; love it because it is God's gift to you. Remember that what you do with your body and the life housed within it is your gift back to God. Reclaim your body and yourself and celebrate life!

MY INWARD JOURNEY

"I will praise thee; for I am fearfully and wonderfully made: marvellous are thy works; and that my soul knoweth right well."

—PSALM 139:14 (KJV)

Inside of you is an intelligent, funny, vivacious, powerful, self-confident woman. Let her out. We are waiting for you.

You are a powerful woman. Using your God-given power, in what three ways can you reclaim your body?

_____

_____

_____

_____

_____

_____

Think of your women friends. Identify the ones you consider powerful. Why? What qualities do they share?

_____

_____

_____

_____

_____

_____

_____

"Teach me O God, to walk in the power of your Spirit. Help me to see what powerful gifts you have placed in me. Amen."

CHAPTER FIVE

Naked and Not Ashamed

When created, Adam and Eve stood before God, naked and unashamed. We need to return to our original place before God. Our bodies, our lives, our sexual drives are natural and healthy components of who we are as God's creation. We should not allow others to define our existence and worth. We are all worth being loved—by ourselves first and then by others. But loved on *our* terms. There are women who have an invisible barrier that blocks them from embracing their sexual selves. For some, it is a misunderstanding about the nature of our sexual selves; for others, there is a barrier of shame and abuse that hinders them from enjoying a healthy sex life.

Shame takes up residence in our lives when we allow someone else to define us or when we give up our power and are unable to get it back because of some sexually traumatic experience—rape, incest, childhood sexual abuse, intimate partner violence, etc. Women who are victims of any form of abuse or experience that has served to hinder their sexual lives can reclaim their sexual power and freedom through facing their fears and overcoming the shame of these experiences. Working through a painful past is the best way to begin the healing process and build up one's self-esteem.

There are thousands of women who are members of a silent sisterhood suffering from an identity crisis. Wonderful women of faith who have been living with guilt and shame because they feel they cannot merge their spiritual selves with their sexual selves. It's like living two lives. The one persona goes to church, is a member of the singles ministry, sings in the gospel choir, belongs to the Women's Fellowship, and mentors young girls in the community. The other persona goes to church, is sexually frustrated, is a member of the singles ministry, and feels guilty when she masturbates, sings in the gospel choir, is desperately trying to find a husband, belongs to the Women's Fellowship, and mentors young girls in the community. Same person, but a divided, tortured existence, searching for healthy, spiritually acceptable ways to satisfy sexual yearnings. There must be reconciliation for a woman with sexual schizophrenia.

Sexual schizophrenia is present in the lives of women who live with a division between their sexual and spiritual identities. They live their lives as fully spiritual women, yet there is a great part of them that is fully sexual. By systematically repressing any form of sexual expression in their lives, they end up exhibiting sexual schizophrenia. The state of sexual schizophrenia is created within women of spirit who try to live under the imposed practices and policies of a male-dominated religious hierarchy. When women of spirit are healed of this malaise, they will experience a release of spiritual power and freedom in their lives. Many women have been taught that they cannot be "good girls" if they give expression to their sexual desires. The church encourages women to express Agape and Phileos, but never Eros unless they are married. Men, on the other hand, are not given such restrictive sexual instructions.

I have always found it interesting that many singles ministries and fellowships in Black churches are overflowing with women of all ages, but there are few if any men in attendance. The singles ministry gives the single women of the church a group to fellowship with in which they do not have to be concerned about being coupled with someone. When I have attended such gatherings, I have noticed a sparse male attendance. I started asking single men at various churches, "Where are you on fellowship nights, and why aren't you at the meetings?" Well, some of the church brothers are out with their friends, some are meeting women at happy hours or nightclubs, and some are just hanging out. Don't act shocked. We're talking about how things really are, not how we think they ought to be. There is a double standard in the church with regard to what is expected of women versus what is expected of men. While some single church women are repressing their sexual desires, waiting for their wedding night, many single church men are not repressing their sexual desires at all. For most men, the idea of abstaining from sex has never entered their minds. They just won't have sex with anyone at their church. Church women are looking for that one special man, and they usually do not date more than one or two men. But brothers, on the other hand, are looking for that one special woman; they will date a number of women until that fateful day of matrimony.

Men and women in the church who have been married and have lost their spouses, whether through death or divorce, have different ideas about their sexual activity now that they are without a spouse. It is silently expected, though it's an imposing expectation, that the women will remain sexually abstinent unless they remarry. However, no such imposition rests upon the grieving widower. It is almost hilarious, the number of women in the church who are eager to console the grieving man and let their intentions be known a few weeks after the funeral. The men mourn their loss and tend to the emotional care of the children. They often talk about their deceased wife; they speak of her fondly, remembering times they spent together, but then the sex issue arises (no pun intended). It is not unusual for me to get a phone call from a widower or to hear, in the midst of a grief-counseling session with a grieving man: "Dr. Newman, when is it appropriate to start going out with women? I'm not used to going this long without sex." I tell them that it is usually frowned upon if a person is seen dating someone before the one-year anniversary of the spouse's funeral, but that they should use as much discretion as possible.

Thomas Moore, a former monk in a Catholic religious order, in his book *The Soul of Sex*, writes, "We have a habit of talking about sex as merely physical, and yet nothing has more soul . . . we separate the body, mind, and emotions as though they were properly contained in individual and unrelated compartments." Moore's observation about the nature of sex is critical to a good understanding of who we are as people, as God's creation. We are not just mind, not just body, not just spirit and soul. Our being is created in such a way that to deny or suppress any part of our makeup is to deny the perfection of God's creation. When my mind is stimulated, my soul and spirit are ignited, and my body gets excited. They coexist to make me who I am—fully, brilliantly, and completely a woman of God!

There is nothing like having a relationship with someone with whom you can share your total self. You may have a friend who is an intellectual companion, one with whom you have the most stimulating conversations, but you are not attracted to him sexually and romantically. Then there is that guy who has your full attention, and he is just as fine as he wants to be. He is an excellent lover and has memorized the *Kama Sutra*, but talking with him is like talking to a box of hair. What is missing is the *soul of sex*.

Have you ever had sex with someone and, while the physical act itself was thrilling, afterward you felt as if there was something missing? Have you ever spent quality time with a person whose very presence excites you—his conversation is always stimulating, and you seem to finish each other's sentences? Haven't you ever wondered what it would be like to make love with someone with whom you share all of these things? This is what I like to call "soulful sex." It is the experience of making love when not only your body is involved in the act, but also your soul, mind, heart, and spirit. There are no barriers present. You are fully in union with another, and the experience of passion transports you both to a new realm of pleasure.

When you have sex with someone, you may enjoy a momentary physical thrill, but without the soul of love, you are only having sex, not making love. Lovemaking involves the offering of total surrender to the beloved, for the purpose of mutual pleasure—this is soulful sex. Soulful sex is not selfish. It desires the fulfillment of the beloved. Soulful sex is not satisfied with "getting some," but with sharing all of oneself with the other. Soulful sex is not the act of "hittin' it and quittin'." Soulful sex lovingly nourishes the beloved with care and affection long after the physical act has ended.

A person can have sex with a total stranger, and it may be physically enjoyable. But a soul that longs for a loving communion with another will only be wounded by having "soulless sex." Soulless sex can be found in the champagne room of the strip club. Soulless sex is the one-night stand. Soulless sex is what women endure because they don't want to be lonely on yet another Friday night. When a woman is looking for love, she will often settle for soulless sex just to have another heartbeat in the house. When women settle for sex when they are looking for love, they are wounding their hearts.

The Greeks have three words for love—*Agape*, *Phileos*, and *Eros*. Agape is that God–human love that is seen in scripture when Jesus says, "Greater love hath no man than this, that a man would lay down his life for his friends" (John 15:13 KJV). Agape is a love that is unconditional, full of grace and mercy. Agape cannot be earned, it is a love that is bestowed upon another as a gift. Phileo is brotherly love. This is love that is shared with those with whom we have a common bond, such as within sororities, families, and organizations. This is why Philadelphia is known as the City of Brotherly Love. We love one another because we have something in common.

Then there is the love expressed as Eros. In today's world, Eros has been corrupted to refer to purely physical sexual acts. But this idea is far from the true nature and role of Eros. Eros is the ingredient in sex that brings intimacy, love, and affection to the sexual encounter. It can be called the "soul of sex." It is Eros that is felt when a couple is making love rather than just experiencing the physical act of sex. Eros brings the emotional bond to the intimate act of sex; it is what we seek in a romantic union with the object of our love. When sex is not only the bodily satisfaction but also a nurturing of one's soul, that is when love is wearing her garments of Eros.

Barriers to Healthy Sex

Many women are unable to enjoy a healthy sex life because of some sexual abuse or domestic violence in their past. These acts have influenced many women's relationships with men, whether the traumas were experienced when the women were children or adults. One in four women report that they have been victims of violence, including domestic violence, intimate partner violence, sexual assault and abuse, rape, and incest. Nonconsensual sex is unhealthy. Any sexual act that injures, degrades, or humiliates another individual is unhealthy. Healthy sex is experienced when two people are feeling good and giving each other pleasure. Everyone experiences sex differently, because we all bring our own past sexual experiences, whether good or bad, to each relationship.

- Rachel links good sex with good caring. She had a wonderful marriage that ended in her husband's death, but the men she meets now don't have the sense of sharing and fun that she likes in a mate. She says that she could not love a person physically without feeling a deep spiritual bond.

- Brenda has been living in darkness all her life; she now lives in the light. She was molested by her uncle for five years. When she was seventeen he moved to another state. Brenda possessed a strong will to overcome this trauma. As an adult she sought therapy and joined a support group in her community. Over a period of time, through carefully developing trusting relationships with men, Brenda now has the ability to heal her past and her sexuality.

A woman's body is sometimes abused even in marriage. The brief but poignant story of Queen Vashti in the Bible's Book of Esther is a good example of this. The story begins in Shushan, the capital city of the Babylonian empire. King Ahasuerus was throwing a seven-day party for the princes and their wives from all 127 provinces of Babylon, from India to Ethiopia. There were gold and silver goblets bejeweled with diamonds, sapphires, rubies, and pearls. The cushions they reclined upon were made from fine silks, and linens threaded with gold. There was plenty of food and drink, and everyone was making merry. Then, on the seventh day, King Ahasuerus sent his servant to get the queen.

Now while the 127 princes and the king were partying in the west wing of the palace, Queen Vashti and the 127 princesses were in the east side of the palace, having a first ladies sort of get-together. When the servant came with the king's request, Queen Vashti responded, in *the* black-woman I-know-you-done-lost-yo'-mind posture, with hands on her hips, "No!" Rev. Dr. Patricia Gould-Champ, pastor of Faith Community Baptist Church in Richmond, Virginia, referred to the king's request as a "booty call." Ahasuerus wanted his wife to entertain his boys with her beautiful body. It is customary for kings to request one or all of their wives to dance and entertain at dinner parties, but this queen was not having any of it. Of course, the king was embarrassed and had to save his reputation in front of the other rulers. For Queen Vashti to refuse her husband's request would be to set a bad example for the other wives. So the king stripped her of her title, took back all that belonged to her as queen, and threw her out of the palace. He then had a beauty contest to search for another wife who would not refuse his every whim and wish.

Like King Ahasuerus, there are many husbands who expect their wives to obey their every sexual wish upon demand. Unfortunately, many women who refuse these sexual requests are raped by their husbands. Recent statistics show that rape is still common in America. Somewhere across the nation, a woman is sexually assaulted every two minutes, according to the U.S. Department of Justice. In the years 1995 and 1996, more than 670,000 women were the victims of rape, attempted rape, or sexual assault.

Nonconsensual sex, even if a prior sexual relationship may have existed, is still rape. Some Christian women don't refuse forced sex from their husbands because their church teaches that wives must submit themselves to their husbands. There needs to be an addendum to the church's class on marriage that gives instructions saying, "When the husband is a substance abuser and/or violent, never submit yourself to him, but pray for him as you call the police."

The women who have been abused, assaulted, stalked, or raped are not the only ones who are profoundly affected by these crimes. The victims' children, family, and friends also suffer from witnessing the violence or hearing the screams or seeing the physical signs of abuse. One of my church members witnessed such violence in her childhood and came to me for pastoral counseling.

Angel is a thirty-four-year-old single woman. She's very active in church, working with the women's ministry and teaching the Young Adult Sunday school class. She sought help because she found herself crying for no apparent reason, and memories from her childhood started bubbling up in her consciousness. I met with her, and after our initial session, I referred her to a psychiatrist for further psychological and emotional assessment, suspecting that she was clinically depressed. The psychiatrist prescribed an antidepressant and agreed to monitor her progress, but Angel wanted to continue her therapy with me.

We met on a weekly basis for nine months. During these sessions she began remembering the pain and fear that had been a part of her childhood. Angel's mother was a waitress at an upscale restaurant in downtown Richmond, Virginia. Her father was a skilled plumber employed by an established company. He made the greater amount of money, but he never seemed to have much of it a few days after payday. It was typical for Angel's father to come home on payday Friday, shower, get dressed up, and go out for the evening. Her mother worked the three-to-ten P.M. shift, and an older woman who had an apartment in the same duplex looked after six-year-old Angel and her four-year-old brother until their mother came home. Angel's mother's wages were not much, but with tips, she earned enough money to buy the kids a few things, contribute to the bills, and buy weekly groceries.

Sometimes Angel's father would not come home. Usually when he got paid he stayed out all night long and came home a couple of days later, drunk, irritable, and broke. He either gambled away his paycheck or spent it all on liquor, women, and good times. He liked playing Big Willie, buying drinks for everyone at the club. If Angel's mother would ask him for money to pay the bills, he wouldn't admit he had none left. An argument would ensue, and things would escalate until Angel's father slapped her mother, then stormed out or fell on the bed to sleep off his drunken stupor. Angel and her little brother would usually hide in the closet or under their bedcovers, trying not to hear their father's angry words and their mother's cries.

No two days were alike for Angel. She never knew what to expect when she came home from elementary school. Either her father would be home, drunk and crying about how bad a father and husband he was, or he would come home drunk and belligerent, and the slightest thing would set him off. Angel's mother always cooked dinner before going to work. One day, Angel's father came home and threw all of the glasses, dishes, pots, and pans on the floor—food and all. He called Angel to the kitchen and told her to clean up the broken dishes and food, all the while ranting and cursing.

Sometimes, Angel would get slapped about when her mother wasn't home and her father needed to vent his anger on someone. Angel would often hang around him when he was home. She didn't care where he'd been or who he'd been with, she was just glad that her daddy was home. Sometimes they watched television together and ate fried bologna sandwiches on white Wonder Bread. But then there were the other times when he didn't seem to recognize Angel and would yell at her as if she were a stranger. Fear was a daily companion for Angel, and she did not know what her future would be like. However, she knew that she would never argue with a man, or ever be with a man who drank alcohol.

Angel was fearful for her mother's life. She would be awake when her mother came home from work and would hear the arguments and hear the awful sound of flesh slapping flesh as her father physically abused her mother. Angel's favorite day of the week was Sunday. On Sunday, she was taken to church, and in Sunday school there was a wonderful teacher who told her that Jesus said, "Suffer the little children to come unto me, and forbid them not: for of such is the kingdom of God" (Mark 10:14 KJV). Angel's teacher told her that God loved her and so did she. She would bring Angel special gifts and talk with her about anything and everything. This spirit-filled woman was an oasis in Angel's wilderness. She planted a seed of God's love in Angel's life that helped her begin a journey toward a Spirit-centered life.

Angel's mother eventually left her husband and moved away with the children. By this time Angel was twelve. To avoid paying child support, Angel's father moved to another state, where he lived with another woman and died, at the age of forty-eight, from cirrhosis of the liver.

Angel has been married and divorced. She said she got married because Eldridge was a nice, handsome man who was soft-spoken and did not drink alcohol. Seven years later they realized that they were strangers to each other. It was during the final stages of their marriage that Angel came to me for counseling and began to accept the fact that she was an ACOA, an Adult Child of an Alcoholic. She joined a twelve-step program to have the support of others with similar backgrounds.

Family violence and abuse are among the most prevalent forms of interpersonal violence against women and young children—both boys and girls. The sexual abuse of a child should never be "just a family matter," but many children are afraid to report an incident to the police because the abuser is often a family friend or relative. According to the Department of Health and Human Services, Administration for Children and Families, Child Maltreatment, in 1995 local child-protective-service agencies identified 126,000 children who were victims of either substantiated or indicated sexual abuse; of these, 75 percent were girls. Nearly 30 percent of child victims were between the ages of four and seven. Approximately one-third of all juvenile victims of sexual abuse cases are children younger than six years of age.

Nicole is a brilliant, vivacious woman in her forties. She owns a natural health food store and is a licensed life coach for women. She shared with me the pain she's lived with and the healing work she's had to do because of sexual abuse she suffered as a child.

My parents divorced when I was about three and since my father didn't give us a dime, my mother had to work twenty-four/seven to support us. One of my "play" uncles, Chuck, was married to a much older woman, and we spent many weekend days at their home. Chuck spent lots of time with my brother and me, and when we were sitting with him on the sofa watching *The Wonderful World of Disney* on TV, he began fondling my vagina. He would sometimes masturbate me to orgasm, with his wife next door cooking dinner in the kitchen. Once we spent the night at their home. I don't remember where my brother slept, but Uncle Chuck asked that I sleep with him and Aunt Clara, in between them. I didn't want to, but he insisted. The next time he wanted to touch me on the sofa, I resisted. He went into the bathroom and called for me to join him. He was nude, with his penis erect. I was four or five years old. He didn't make me touch it, but he told me with a sneer that when I grew up I'd beg for it. I remember the musky smell of his private parts, which were level with my face.

Nicole is now just beginning to heal from this experience. She has been doing a lot of spiritual, emotional, and healing work—including forgiving "Uncle" Chuck, who died an early and painful death when Nicole was an adolescent.

There are thousands of women just like Nicole who have suffered childhood sexual abuse. These women's sexual self-esteem was scarred early in life, and they continue to carry these scars with them into adulthood. Many do seek counseling and begin the arduous task of revisiting the horrific experience, some at the risk of "rewounding" themselves. It is because of the barrier of an unhealthy introduction to sex that some women are unable to enjoy a healthy sexual relationship with another person, or even with themselves.

How wonderful it would have been if the church that Nicole attended had a youth pastor or someone who had been trained to oversee a safe place for a child or young person to talk about sensitive issues and receive help. There are faith-based sex education curriculums that teach adults how to talk to young people about sex and how to create an atmosphere in a church that conveys, "This is a safe place to talk about sex." (See the "Resources" section at the end of this book.) Women like Nicole suffer from a myriad of issues that relate to their sexual abuse as a child. As Nicole described herself:

Like many people who have experienced child sexual abuse, I suffer from low self-esteem, the inability to trust,

and difficulty asserting myself properly in personal situations. Like many women with similar histories, I learned
early on how to be popular with men and the power of sex
withheld or granted. I also learned to compartmentalize
my mind and body so that I could be completely detached
during sex. I knew I was "good in bed," and while I was
never promiscuous, I had sex with guys sometimes just because they wanted it and I was not able to say no!

In *The Washington Post*, July 30, 2001, in an article titled "Sex
Abuse at Church Shatters a Family," David A. Fahrenthold de-
tailed a horrific story, exposing a popular Black Baptist Church in
which a deacon sexually molested a young boy. The church leaders were silent when they found out. At the age of eight, the boy
broke down crying and told his older brother that when he was
five and six he had been abused by a deacon. The deacon, a forty-
five-year-old man who had joined the church ten years earlier,
turned out to be a convicted child molester, having pleaded guilty
in 1989 in D.C. Superior Court to molesting his nine-year-old
stepdaughter. At the time he was hired, the church was in the
midst of searching for a new pastor, and the deacon board had been
in charge of all operations. Later, when interviewed by the press,
the pastor emeritus who ordained the man into the position of deacon said, "As a people of faith, we don't require a checkup on people [about] what their past life has been . . . we welcome them with
love." The pastor emeritus went on to say, "He had a special interest in the bus ministry."

The deacon was given the job of picking up and dropping off
children each Sunday. He began doting on this one boy when the
boy was five. He would give the boy money for being good in

church. He asked the boy's mother if the child could stay after church and help him clean up after the service, and she agreed. The mother saw this as an opportunity for her young son to be influenced by a good male leader of the church, a good role model. For the next several months, the boy was sexually molested by the deacon. One day the deacon brought the boy home very late, and the mother discontinued the relationship. After the mother found out about the abuse, she and her family left the church in D.C. and joined another church in Maryland.

In late 1998 the mother told the pastor of her new church what had happened. He set up a meeting with the deacons of her former church, and the deacon admitted that he had abused the boy. The deacon board assured the mother that the man would no longer have contact with children, but last year the mother found out that he was once again working with kids. She decided to press charges. He was charged with four acts of sexual abuse and sentenced to two to ten years in prison.

Why was he allowed to continue working with children? Why didn't the deacon board support this mother in pressing charges against the man when his crime was discovered? These things happen because good, well-intentioned people keep silent, and this kind of silence in the Black church is killing the black community. We cannot afford to allow shame to silence us. When the church finds its voice on issues of sexuality, and sex is no longer a taboo, then and only then can the church help victims of incest, rape, domestic violence, and sexual abuse who sit in the church's pews on cushioned seats Sunday after Sunday, seeking the peace of God.

It is important that our culture and society educate our children about sexuality—what children should know and when they should know it are very important. By the time a girl is four, five, or six years old, she should know the terms for all sexual body parts. She should know the difference between girls and boys, women and men. She should know the truth about where babies come from, and not be told the old stories about the stork and the cabbage patch (I didn't eat cabbage for years—I thought there were baby parts in the pot). Girls should be able to talk about their bodies with their mothers at home. Most important, they should understand that their bodies belong to them and that they have a right to say no to unwanted touching. This is also an excellent time to begin sharing with young girls the importance of good hygiene and maintaining good health.

Preadolescent and adolescent girls can begin talking about the physical changes they can expect in their bodies, including breast growth, the appearance of body hair, and the onset of menstruation. It is important for young girls to know that these are all natural and good signs of their maturation. This is also the crucial time to begin talking about the sacredness of their bodies and to give them an understanding of human sexuality and the responsibilities that accompany this gift. Of course, discussing the possibility of pregnancy, choices in contraception, and the prevention of sexually transmitted diseases are critical components of sex talk at this age.

PHYSICAL ABUSE

Domestic violence or physical abuse in the lives of women is significantly linked to sex. Whether women are sexually harassed at work, beaten in their home, or bearing the psychological wounds

NAKED AND NOT ASHAMED

from childhood abuse, sex is interwoven in the fabric of their experience. All abuse, emotional and psychological, impacts women's
spiritual health and wellness. A slap in the face is a blow to her
self-esteem. The resulting pain wounds and damages the victim.
Many victims of intimate partner violence experience sex after
the violent act as a form of apology. The sexual feelings experienced momentarily disguise the cruel and shameful acts of violence that lie beneath the relationship. Some have said, "There's
no sex better than make-up sex." There is no amount of sex that
can excuse or make up for sexual or physical abuse.

Physical abuse is usually recurrent and escalates in both fre-
quency and severity. Although most assaults on women do not
result in death, they do result in physical injury and severe emotional distress. Physical injuries are the most tangible manifesta-
tions of domestic violence, yet frequently they are not reported by
women and go unrecognized by the professionals who are man-
dated to intervene.

Psychological abuse of women is underestimated, trivialized,
and at times difficult to define. Psychological abuse has been reported by abused women to be as damaging as physical battering
because of its impact on their self-image. It often precedes or ac-
companies physical abuse, but it may occur by itself. Sexual assault consists of a range of behaviors that may include pressured
sex when victims do not desire sex, coerced sex by manipulation
or threat, physically forced sex, or sexual assault accompanied by
violence. Victims may be forced or coerced to perform a type of
sex act they do not desire, or at a time they do not want it. For
some battered victims this sexual violation is profound and difficult to discuss.

Emotional abuse represents a method of control that may

consist of verbal attacks and humiliations, including repeated verbal attacks against the victim's worth as an individual or role as a parent, family member, coworker, friend, or community member. The verbal attacks often emphasize the victim's vulnerabilities. Isolation occurs when perpetrators try to control victims' time, activities, and contact with others. Perpetrators may accomplish this through interfering with supportive relationships, creating barriers to normal activities (such as taking away the car keys or locking the victim in the home), and lying or distorting what is real to gain psychological control.

Economic abuse is when perpetrators control access to all of the victims' resources, such as time, transportation, food, clothing, shelter, insurance, and money. Perpetrators may interfere with victims' ability to become self-sufficient, and insist on controlling all of the finances. When the victim leaves the violent relationship, the perpetrator may use economics as a way to maintain control or force a return. There are women who are victims of economic abuse sitting in the pew next to you every Sunday.

Brokenness and pain from our past conceal the gifts of hope and transformation that God has for us. Transformation is the key to our new beginnings. It is not always obvious at first, but time reveals it to us. My sister, Connie, makes wonderful things out of glass. She makes sun catchers, stained-glass window designs, and prayer boxes. One day I visited with Connie, and, as usual, glass was everywhere. On the floor were a few panes of pink, purple, and green glass that had apparently fallen off the counter and broken. I was upset because they were broken, but Connie said, "Oh, that's okay. I use the broken pieces to create a new picture or design for a new window."

Life is like that. God can use the broken pieces of our past to create a new design for our future. "We know that all things work together for good for those who love God" (Romans 8:28). If you are a victim of sexual or physical abuse, today is a good day to get help and get out of that no-win situation. In the back of this book in the "Resources" section, there are agencies that you can call for help.

MY INWARD JOURNEY

He that dwelleth in the secret place of the most High shall abide under the shadow of the Almighty. I will say of the Lord, He is my refuge and my fortress; my God; in him will I trust.

—PSALM 91:1–2 (KJV)

Have you ever been naked and ashamed? What was going on, and how did you feel?

_____

_____

_____

_____

_____

_____

_____

Stand in front of a mirror, naked, and begin to thank God for parts of your body. Example: "God, I thank you that I have full breasts. They remind me that I'm able to feed a child."

_____

_____

_____

_____

_____

_____

_____

Have you ever experienced any form of abuse? Get a separate journal and begin remembering the experience. Jot down what you saw, what you heard, what you felt. If you are still broken because of this, seek help and healing now. Look in the "Resources" section of this book and call someone.

CHAPTER SIX

From Celibate to Celebrate

Now that you've begun this journey of honesty about how your sexual feelings fit into your life as a woman of faith, what are you going to do about it? What are the options that lie before you as a woman of a sensuous and spiritual nature? Well, before you throw caution to the wind and jump in feetfirst (or is it bottoms up?), let's take a little time to examine what our choices are in the realm of sexual expression. There is not any one particular answer to this question; it is up to you how you choose to live your life.

I already know that many women may be uncomfortable about focusing upon what kind of sexual lifestyle they want—but *I* know you want one, and *you* know you want one, so let's have a heart-to-heart about where you fit in. Several years ago, I was invited to teach a workshop at a very conservative Black Baptist church in Washington, D.C. They gave me the title of my seminar, Sex and the Single Christian. The seminar was on a Saturday morning from nine A.M. to noon. I arrived at the church, entered the large meeting room, and saw about eighty faces looking back at me. There were men and women between the ages of twenty-five and sixty-five, all waiting to spend three hours talking about sex and the single Christian.

I began, "Good morning, I am Reverend Susan Newman; please turn with me to First Corinthians, chapter seven, verse one." I read: "It is good for a man not to touch a woman." Then I closed my Bible and said, "Let us stand for closing prayer." They looked at me as if I'd lost my mind. I asked, "What's wrong? There's nothing else to say or do today, because I know you are all going to sit here and pretend that you're doing nothing but praising the Lord under the sheets at night. I'm sure we all have something else we can do with three hours on a Saturday morning. But, we can have a very productive time together if we can agree to operate within certain assumptions. First, let's say, for the sake of our purposes today, that you are either involved in a sexually intimate relationship now, or you hope to meet someone here today who may tickle your fancy, or you are looking for me to affirm whatever sexual behavior you're involved in already. If we all agree to operate from one of these assumptions, then we can talk about responsible sexuality. We can examine what happens when you are sexually intimate with someone who is not your spouse, or you are sexually intimate with someone, but the relationship is not a committed monogamous relationship."

Everyone in the room agreed to operate under these assumptions for our remaining time. They agreed to stop pretending that sex was not a problem for them as single Christians. They admitted that they loved the Lord, but they missed the physical intimacy of another person. They agreed to engage in an honest dialogue about the consequences of having sex with someone when there is no commitment, no monogamy, no marriage. Everyone took off their I'm-happy-in-Jesus-alone mask and began talking about their sexual desires and frustrations when trying to be celibate. The remaining time was spent sharing stories about game playing, dishonesty in relationships, how sexual intimacy without a personal commitment is not the best choice for many, and the importance of having a partner who is spiritually compatible with you. We had a productive exchange of ideas, after clearing the air of our pretenses and sexual facades as church people.

On another occasion, I facilitated a retreat with a group of women from a church in the Washington, D.C., area. During the retreat, about twelve women sat around in my hotel suite talking about their beliefs related to sex, the church, and relationships. Each woman had something significant to share that reflects the feelings and thoughts of many women.

Tammy is a very attractive, thirty-two-year-old black woman. While we were discussing celibacy, Tammy shared this:

> It wasn't in my spirit and I wasn't going to say, "I'm celibate and I'm not going to have sex." But when I made a conscious decision to be celibate, it wasn't so much that it was a religious thing, but I wanted to have sex with the person I was going to marry—we would have to be at the point of marriage or very close. I don't want to give that special part of myself to just anyone. I don't want to be spiritually connected to a man that I've had sex with if we are not getting married. I see how I act [after being

sexually intimate with someone]. I was with the same guy for six years, and I see what it did to me when we broke up and tried to get back together and we had sex. Once I found out he was having sex with other people, I lost my mind. How could he share that with someone else?

Tammy's experience is similar to that of many women. She chose to refrain from sexual intercourse until she was in a relationship with someone whom she thought she'd marry. For Tammy, sexual intimacy bonds her with her partner. In the Book of Genesis, it says "Now the man knew his wife Eve, and she conceived and bore Cain" (4:1). It's interesting that in the scriptures, the term *knew* is a synonym for sexual intercourse. For many, there is a knowledge that is shared between two people who have sex. Tammy called this a "special part" of herself, and said that she did not take sharing it with another lightly. Unfortunately, although Tammy felt this way, her boyfriend did not. When she found out he was sexually active with another woman, she "lost her mind." She did not like how it made her feel. It is important to choose a partner who believes as you do—someone with values that are compatible with yours.

Some people engage in recreational sex. They do not make commitments and don't want to be questioned about who else they are dating. Being clear about what each person expects out of a relationship is crucial. Even though Tammy was thinking "forever," her boyfriend was thinking "for now."

Lisa is twenty-eight years old, very quiet and serious when speaking about sex and the importance of knowing the right time to be intimate with a partner.

As little girls, we're told that this is a gift [your body] and don't give it to anybody unless you want to give it to them. When a lot of women give themselves to men, they feel like this is something only you yourself can give to them, and, beyond emotions, you are giving something that you cherish and you expect him to cherish it as much as you do. But most men don't; sex is just an act. Women bring their heart and soul to the bed, but most men just bring their body. Then I realize, now that I've done this with you—I'm vulnerable.

Lisa echoes the sentiments of thousands of women. When some women have sex with a man, their heart and soul are involved. For many of these women, they are in love after having sex, they feel a bond with this man, they've given themselves fully in the sexual act. Unfortunately, for many men it was just sex. There is a double moral standard that our culture nourishes in regard to the expectations of sexual behavior of men and women. Women are supposed to be chaste and virginal until they are married. But men in our culture are expected to be virile and sexually active. That's why marriage is seen by many as giving up one's freedom.

Men are expected to sow their wild oats while they're single. Some brothers today are called "big baller, shot caller" or "playa, playa." For these brothers, they feel that it is their right to date more than one woman and "get their freak on" as often as possible, without any repercussions from an already existing relationship. And if one of their lady friends objects, the usual response is, "Don't hate the playa, hate the game!" Well, I hate all of it. This same brother wants to do his thing and wants a "good girl" to be a wife and the mother of his children. For a great number of men, they still play the game even after they are married. This is when sex becomes dangerous.

Don't be Boo-Boo the Fool when choosing your partner. Multiple sex partners is like playing Russian roulette: you never know which shot will be the lethal one. When considering the choices and consequences of being intimately involved, women not only have to consider whether or not their man is dating other women, but whether he is dating men as well. Some men consider themselves bisexual. Some don't consider themselves bisexual, they say they're just "doin' it on the down-low." Whatever you call it, it's low-down to be sexually intimate with more than one person and lie to your partners and yourself about what's really going on.

When E. Lynn Harris's first book, *Invisible Life*, hit the book-stores, I got my copy and felt as if I were reading about people I knew. I read the disclaimer in the front of the book: "This novel is a work of fiction. Names, characters, places, and incidents either are the product of the author's imagination or are used fictitiously. Any resemblance to actual persons, living or dead, events, or locales is entirely coincidental." In the words of Gomer Pyle, "Shazam!" I went to school, work, and church with people who matched the products of Harris's imagination. One of Harris's acclaimed characters, Basil Henderson, is every woman's dream and nightmare. A fine, successful, sexy black man who is just as savvy in the boardroom as the bedroom, Basil operates on the "down-low." He's sexually intimate with both men and women. Basil whets his appetite with young men with the physique of a Greek god, then goes out later the same night hunting for some new honeys.

Well, Basil may be a fictional character in the book, but he is real life for a whole lot of folks. It has been said, "You cannot judge a book by its cover." That's why it is critical for women considering sexual intimacy with someone to first consider the consequences. The wise ones of our culture have said, "Every good-bye ain't gone, every shut eye ain't sleep, and everybody laughing ain't tickled." In other words, things (and people) are not always what they seem. If your heart is all aflutter for someone, take time to get to know him. If he is worth your sharing your love with, then he will be willing to wait for your consent.

I asked one guy, "How many girlfriends do you have?" He answered, "None." I said, "I'm sure *you think* that you have none, but how many women are there who *think* they are your girlfriend?" "About four," he replied. This is when irresponsible sex can be dangerous. When choosing to be sexually intimate with anyone, you have to ask questions, take time to get to know the person, consider the consequences, and do all of this before you get all hot and bothered!

CHOICES

Our lives are filled with choices: Paper or plastic? Can or bottle? Supersize your order? Unleaded or leaded? Smoking or nonsmoking? Aisle or window? Friend of the bride or of the groom? Cream or sugar? VHS or DVD? Black-and-white or color? Cash, check, or charge? All of life presents choices to us, and God has gifted us with the power of rational thought, deduction, intuitive thinking, and a wonderful intellect.

Although we can observe the actions of others and learn from their successes and failures, ultimately we must make our own decisions based upon what life has taught us. We make life decisions using our God-given intellect and spirit. We choose what makes us feel like healthy, whole, natural women. After we have attended all the seminars, conferences, and lectures, and after we have read every book, memorized every principle, and viewed every video, we must make choices based upon what feels life-nurturing to us. Many of our decisions are not that drastically different from those of others, but there are slight differences, and we have to be true to who we are. One of my friends does not like to sleep under sheets. She doesn't mind the bottom sheet, but she will not use the top sheet; she prefers sleeping under a quilt. I, on the other hand, love sheets. I don't need quilts, bedspreads, blankets, or comforters—just sheets. Except, of course, for when it gets cold. Then I want the sheets, the quilt, the bedspread, the blanket, *and* the comforter. It's all about individual preferences.

I know it's hard to break out on one's own and do things differently from the crowd. I can remember my mother's response when, as a teenager, I wanted to do something because "all my friends are doing it!" Momma would reply, "If your friends jumped off a cliff, would you jump off, too?" So don't be just like someone else, be who you are, with all your uniqueness. Let what others do influence you to *think* about how *you* feel about a particular issue, and then make your own decision based upon what feels right, whole, sane, and natural to your spirit.

One of the most difficult things for many people to accomplish in life is self-trust. We simply don't trust ourselves. We put our trust in others, but not ourselves. Think about it. Every day we put our trust in some of the most untrustworthy things and people. Yet, we've been with ourselves for our whole lives and we don't *trust us*. We will get on an airplane that some unknown people made and let a strange crew take us thirty thousand feet into the sky. We trust that the stranger in the cockpit knows what he's doing. But did you see his credentials? Was her flight school diploma on the cockpit wall? Did he wash down that breakfast burrito with a little of "the recipe" in his coffee? We don't know, but we're just a'ridin' and a'trustin'.

And we believe that if the plane malfunctions and we begin to fall thirty thousand feet, that if we fasten our seat belt, put on our oxygen mask, and hold on to our seat cushion, we'll be all right. We trust the airline attendants. They said we would be all right if we followed their instructions. There must be some drugs in that package of peanuts and pretzel mix they serve, 'cause we calm right on down and are content with a thimble of soda and gooby-dusted nuts. Do you trust this? I find it hard to trust anyone small enough to walk up and down such a narrow aisle, carrying a tray of drinks thirty thousand feet in the air without falling into some-one's lap. But we just a'ridin' and a'trustin'.

Okay, maybe you can't relate to flying. You're sitting there thinking, "That's why I don't fly." Well, you probably ride in an elevator every day. We trust those elevators made by the Otis Company. We will get into a small steel box suspended by a few cables, and trust that it will take us safely to the thirty-eighth floor. While we are standing there, concentrating on not looking into the eyes of the other people, we stare up at the lights or read the certificate on which some stranger has signed his name, assur-ing us that this steel box suspended by a few cables is able to safely deliver a thousand pounds (no one weighed us before we got in) to the thirty-eighth floor. We just a'ridin' and a'trustin'. Who is "Otis" anyway?

Yet, we often don't trust our own decisions and judgments about our individual lives. Etta James recorded a song that says, "Trust in me, in all you do." I imagine our spirit singing this song to our heart and mind. As women of spirit, we consciously nurture our relationship with God. We seek God's peace, love, and power in our lives daily. When we are facing a moment of decision, we need to realize that it is through our God-centered spirit that we receive guidance. As we learn to love God with our whole selves—heart, mind, body, and soul—we will learn to trust our own decisions.

Dr. Lawrence N. Jones, the dean at Howard University Divinity School when I was a seminarian, always used to tell us to "trust in the trustworthiness of God." If you are living in the presence of Spirit, then trust that Spirit has gifted you with all you need to live, breathe, and move through life. Begin to make life-nurturing decisions and trust them. Does it feel natural and empowering? Does it feel sane to you? Is this the choice that allows your inner child to stop crying, seeking, and searching for reassurance, and that enables your inner child to lie down in comfort and peace? Then you've made a life-nurturing decision—trust it.

Why are we unable to trust ourselves? I believe that the twin tools that diminish our lives are doubt and discouragement. They are subtle, yet powerful adversaries. Many of us can hear ten positive things about ourselves and one negative thing, and it is the one negative that we cradle to our breast and feed off of daily. Each morning, we bathe in doubt and clothe ourselves in discouragement. When people bring more of it into our presence, we receive it as if we deserve it and gladly adorn ourselves with this raiment that robs us of our dignity. We are constantly seeking acceptance and affirmation that we are all right just the way we are, but then doubt reminds us of some terrible mistake we've made in the past. And so we move through life carrying this heavy baggage that diminishes us daily. We can't move forward toward making new and wonderful memories because we are so weighed down by the baggage of the past. Well, it's time to unpack your bags and move forward!

A RESPONSIBLE SEXUAL LIFE

Let's look at some of the issues women may encounter when they are sexually intimate with a partner with whom there is no established relationship or commitment. Women feel vulnerable after being sexually intimate with a man. Women and men think and feel differently about various things; they have different expectations and values. Consider the concept of *time*, for instance. There is *boy time* and *girl time*. Let's look at Jennifer and Jeffrey. They meet at a city-wide, church-sponsored, singles retreat. Then Jennifer and Jeffrey talk on the phone several times during the week and set a date for the weekend. Within a two-week period, Jeff takes her to lunch, to a jazz club for dinner and dancing, and to a gospel concert. They like each other. They share a wonderful kiss and embrace the night they go to the jazz club. She's started telling her girlfriends about him. He's cute, has a good job, drives a sporty car, and makes her laugh. Unlike a lot of guys, Jeff has not tried to force the issue of sex.

Jeff likes Jennifer, too. She's pretty and smart, and never seems bored when he's talking about what's important to him. His best friend, Donald, teases him about getting too serious with Jennifer. Jeffrey has always dated three women at a time, while Jennifer always gives her full attention to one man at a time. Unfortunately, she zeros in too soon, seeing every new date as husband material. But Jeffrey is nowhere near ready to get married.

Their fourth week dating, Jennifer invites Jeffrey for a home-cooked meal at her apartment on Friday night. She pulls out all the stops, trying to get him to imagine what it would be like to be married to her. She's a good cook and throws down in the kitchen that day. They share a dinner of smothered chicken and gravy, mashed potatoes, tossed salad, green peas with pearl onions (his favorite), and corn muffins. The dinner is topped off with pound cake and strawberry slices, accented with whipped cream. He is impressed and pleased that she took the time to prepare such a meal for him. After dinner they go for a walk in a nearby park to help their dinner digest. Holding hands, Jennifer tells Jeffrey how special she feels when she's with him. Jeffrey says, "That's because you are special." He pulls a small box out of his pocket, and she takes it with her heart in her throat. Inside is a pair of diamond stud earrings. Jennifer throws her arms around his neck and squeals, "Thank you!" Jeffrey says, "Well, we met a month ago, and I wanted to give you something."

They return to her apartment and one thing leads to another; they enjoy each other sexually for the rest of the night. Jennifer is up early the next morning, cooking breakfast and humming to herself, when Jeffrey comes into the kitchen, fully dressed and ready to leave. He walks toward her, saying, "I had a great time last night, and you are so-o-o-o-o hot! But I got to take my mother to the mall and a bunch of other places." As he leaves, he says, "I'll give you a call in a couple of days."

Now, in *girl time* a couple of days is *two* days. It's Saturday morning when he says this, so a couple of days means that he should call no later than Monday at noon. But in *boy time*, a couple of days is anywhere from two days to two weeks! Jennifer doesn't hear from Jeffrey until Friday around four P.M. She's spent the last five days agonizing over why he has not called. "I shouldn't have had sex with him; now he's gotten what he wanted and he's gone!" "I thought he loved me; he gave me diamond stud earrings." "I wasn't expecting any of this; we didn't even use a condom." "I could have herpes, syphilis, or worst yet—AIDS!" "I thought he was different; he's a Christian man, sweet, and now this."

Jennifer goes on a round-trip guilt trip all week because she had sex with Jeffrey and he has not called her. He's not the first guy with whom this has happened, but he was the first guy who was a Christian, and she thought he would be different. She was wrong. Unfortunately, Jennifer's situation is not unique. Men and women meet, date, and spend wonderful days and evenings together, but never say what they are expecting out of the relationship. Again, we find it difficult to be honest, but honesty is the only way. If one person is looking for a commitment and the other isn't, then hearts will break. If we say that we are spiritual men and women, then we should treat each other with a greater respect and just put our cards on the table from the beginning. Once you're in the bed and bells and whistles are going off, it's dangerous for a brother to say to a sister who's looking for commitment, "I thought we was just kickin' it." All of a sudden the music of an old school song can be heard in the background: "It's a thin line between love and hate."

In the movie *When Harry Met Sally*, two acquaintances from college move to New York, become friends, and share the highs and lows of each other's relationships. They do everything together; they share the intimate details of their love affairs, and they share hopes of someday meeting "the one." One night they have sex with each other. They both have difficulty dealing with how sex has now totally shifted the paradigm of their friendship. She was feeling warm and fuzzy afterward; he enjoyed it too much and needed to flee. Three weeks later, at their best friends' wedding, they confront each other about it. Sally says, "Why do you act as if it didn't mean anything?" Harry replies, "Why do you act as if it means everything?" She slaps him and walks away.

In affairs of the heart, the important thing is "communication, communication, communication." But most brothers don't want to talk, and if you keep insisting on it, and they want to walk, well, as hard as it may be, and as fine as he may be, politely show him the door. If he's not willing to talk about relationship expectations and what's important to you now, know that down the road it will not get any better. You are a woman of spirit, and you will be off balance sharing your time and treasure with an unbalanced brother. If he is not a Spirit-centered man, then it's like trying to talk to someone from another planet. Don't share your body with anyone with whom you have not already shared your spirit.

God is so central to our sexual natures that even an atheist cannot experience an orgasm without calling on the name of the Lord. I am not aware of anyone who has ever, in the midst of passion, cried out, "Oh Buddha!" or "Oh Mohammad," but invariably one will be heard to say, "Oh God!" That is because, despite what we are taught about sex being sinful, for women sexual activity is *sacred activity*, according to Dr. John Kinney, dean of the Virginia Theological Seminary in Richmond, Virginia. As women, we are cocreators with God. When we engage in sexual intercourse, the possibility of creating a new life and incubating and nurturing that life for nine months is a sacred activity that women share with God. We are able to birth new life into the world. Therefore, it is critical that we take care of our sexual selves and behave responsibly with our bodies and spirits.

Accepting responsibility for your sexual health is critical in this age of HIV (human immunodeficiency virus) and AIDS (autoimmune deficiency syndrome) and other STDs (sexually transmitted diseases). It is important to be assertive and clearly state your desire to practice safe sex. This is a discussion that you both should have way before the arrival of any moments of mounting passion. Always make sure you have a condom; do not rely on your partner to have one. Some may think, "If I carry a condom, then I subconsciously plan to have sex." Not true. If you carry a condom, you are being honest with yourself that, in this age of mounting cases of HIV among heterosexual African American women between the ages of twenty-four and forty-five, you refuse to become another statistic. My mother taught me that it is better to have it and not need it, than to need it and not have it. Of course, Mom was talking about money, but I have found her advice on this to be universal in application.

WOMEN AND HIV

As the HIV/AIDS epidemic continues, more women are becoming infected with HIV, the virus that causes AIDS. Women, like men, can get HIV infection through sex and blood-to-blood contact, which can occur as a result of needle sharing. Because the number of women who are infected is increasing, it is important to know how to prevent HIV infection. As women, you can take responsibility for protecting your own health. Symptoms vary from person to person, and they do not necessarily indicate HIV infection. Only a test can tell if someone has HIV; only a doctor can diagnose AIDS.

The most common ways that HIV is spread are:

- having vaginal, oral, or anal sex with someone who has HIV
- sharing needles or syringes with someone who has HIV
- During pregnancy, childbirth, or breast-feeding, when a mother with HIV passes it to her baby

HIV is not spread through everyday social activity. This means that hugging, touching, cuddling, kissing, and massaging do not spread HIV, as long as there is no contact with an infected person's blood, semen, vaginal fluid, or breast milk.

Not having sex is the only sure way to avoid sexual transmission of HIV. But, if you decide to have sex, you can reduce your risk of infection in several ways:

- Be in a committed monogamous relationship, whereby you are having sex with only one partner who does not have HIV.
- When having sex, use a latex condom every time, which greatly reduces your risk of infection.
- Avoid contact with your partner's blood, semen, or vaginal fluid.
- For oral sex with a man, use a condom without spermicide or lubricants (they come in flavors).
- For oral sex with a woman, use a dental dam as a barrier to vaginal fluids (Saran Wrap serves the same purpose).

I know it may be a little uncomfortable for some folks to talk about or even read about these things, but it is this kind of information that will save your life. As long as we are being honest with ourselves, we can change our behavior to reduce our risk of any sexually transmitted disease or infection. Even if you are not sexually intimate with anyone, you may still need to know this information in order to help someone else.

Self-Pleasuring

Most of us were discouraged from masturbating as children. Masturbation is a normal sexual activity that does not result in any kind of emotional, physical, or spiritual harm. Some do not choose to masturbate. That, too, is a healthy choice. Some ministers teach that masturbation is an evil tool of the devil, calling it the "Sin of Onan," referring to a passage of scripture in Genesis.

Judah, one of Israel's twelve patriarchs, chose a wife, Tamar, for his eldest son, Er. The Bible says Er was wicked in the eyes of God, and the Lord put him to death. According to the customs of the Hebrew people, when a woman was widowed, she then became the property and wife of the next male relative of her husband. So Judah gave Tamar to his next eldest son, Onan. He instructed Onan to obey the Levitical Law of bearing a son for his deceased brother, saying, "Go in to your brother's wife and perform the duty of a brother-in-law to her; raise up offspring for your brother."

Onan knew that the child would be considered Er's son and not his, so whenever he had sex with Tamar, he withdrew himself before ejaculating and "spilled his semen on the ground." Thus, not obeying the Levitical Law of bearing seed for his brother, Onan displeased God and was killed as was his brother before him. By this time, Judah suspected that there was something terribly wrong with this woman, Tamar. He'd lost two sons, and the only thing they had had in common, besides being siblings, was the fact that they had both married her. Judah began seeing Tamar as a black widow spider. Judah knew that his boys had been all right, so something was wrong with this gal! Instead of giving Tamar to his youngest and sole remaining son, Shelah, Judah told his daughter-in-law, "Remain a widow in your father's house until my son Shelah grows up." Judah was afraid that he would lose Shelah as well. So Tamar went to live in her father's house.

A few years passed and Judah's wife died; after a period of

mourning, Judah hooked up with his friend Hirah, and they went to a sheep-shearing convention in a nearby town. This was Judah's first time away since his wife died. He ain't been with no woman for ages, and you know some men ain't used to going a long time without some lovin'. So he and his boy Hirah go out for a night of wine, women, and song in Timnah (a forerunner to Las Vegas).

Well, someone told Tamar that her father-in-law was going to Timnah for a little R and R. She realized that he wasn't going to let her marry Shelah, yet she knew she had to raise up seed for her late husband. Tamar changed from her widow's clothes to prostitute's garb and went and sat outside the gates of Timnah. When Judah saw her, he wanted to have sex with her.

> She said, "What will you give me, that you may come in to me?" He answered, "I will send you a kid from the flock." And she said, "Only if you give me a pledge, until you send it." He said, "What pledge shall I give you?" She replied, "Your signet and your cord, and the staff that is in your hand." So he gave them to her, and went in to her, and she conceived by him. Then she got up and went away, and taking off her veil she put on the garments of her widowhood. [Later that week, Judah sent Hirah back to Timnah with the sheep to exchange for his things, but Hirah could not find her, and no one in the town knew her.] About three months later Judah was told, "Your daughter-in-law Tamar has played the whore; moreover she is pregnant as a result of whoredom." [Judah was outraged because Tamar had brought sin and shame upon his family name and the name of his deceased son, Er.] And Judah said, "Bring her out, and let her be burned." As she

was being brought out, she sent word to her father-in-law, "It was the owner of these who made me pregnant." And she said, "Take note, please, whose these are, the signet and the cord and the staff." Then Judah acknowledged them and said, "She is more in the right than I, since I did not give her to my son Shelah" (Genesis 38:6–26).

So you see, the sin of Onan is not about masturbation at all. It's about Onan's refusal to fulfill the Levite Law and procreate with his dead brother's wife. Onan does not masturbate to avoid procreation. He "spilled his seed on the ground" to avoid impregnating Tamar.

Some religious leaders believe and teach that self-pleasuring is wrong; however, I hope that, as you are reassessing your beliefs and attitudes, you will open your spirit and mind to the natural act of pleasuring yourself. How can you share with your lover what will arouse and please you if you do not know firsthand for yourself?

I prefer to use the term *self-pleasuring*; it sounds much less technical than *masturbation*. We are created to receive pleasure from our own bodies. However, it is important to know that, sexually, we are more than just genitals. Our entire body can be sensual and pleasing—if we take time to fully discover our sexual selves. Think about how pleasing it is to feel a soft kiss upon your forehead, the stroke of a hand on your arm, or warm breath next to your ear. All of you is sensual.

What pleases you? Plan to spend an evening alone, getting in touch with *you*. Remember when you first met that special someone? Everywhere you went, you bought things that would please your beloved. Well, now I'm asking you to do things that will please you.

- Buy your favorite flowers and put them in a beautiful vase.
- Prepare your favorite meal. Play music that makes you "feel like a natural woman."
- Get a full-body deep-tissue massage.
- Sleep on silk or satin sheets.
- Burn various scented oils for relaxation.
- Look at your body as if it were fine jewelry.

Exploring your body through self-touch is another way to become more aware of what gives you sexual pleasure. Women should find out which sensations bring them the most enjoyment. It is good to know for yourself, before you try to share this information with your lover.

Dr. June Dobbs-Butts, noted African American sex therapist, has said, The body's largest sex organ lies between the ears, not between the legs. Surprising, isn't it? We've been socialized to believe that sexual satisfaction is greatly dependent upon the size of certain body parts. How many times have you heard women whispering about the size of a man's shoes or hands? We don't know where certain ideas originated, but we can all quote, "It's not the size of the ship, but the motion of the ocean. . . . It's not the size of the engine, but the skill of the engineer." I can't count the number of times I've heard women describing the wonderful attributes of a new boyfriend by saying, "He's bow-legged!"

There are different things that will "float one's boat," sexually speaking. However, these stimulating messages are fed into our brain through our five senses: sight, smell, touch, hearing, and taste. All of these sensory stimulants excite us through our brain, and when the brain has received enough excitement for our own personal threshold, we thus experience an orgasm. We are

God-gifted to please ourselves, independent of another person. Yes, it is wonderful to share this experience with another, but there are times when we may choose to be alone. Our sensual experiences are not solely dependent upon our genitals. The truth is, women have choices. They may choose to marry or live their lives fully, brilliantly, and completely as single women in a monogamous relationship. Whether a woman chooses to have a loving partner to experience the joys of sexual intimacy, or chooses to use all of her God-given senses to bring pleasure into her own personal realm of enjoyment and fulfillment—it is her body, her life, her choice.

CELIBACY

Celibacy is more than abstaining from sexual intercourse, it is choosing to abstain from sexual intercourse when there is no healthy, loving, monogamous, committed relationship present in your life. Celibacy is a wonderful sexual preference, but a choice that should be made in joy and peace, not in resolve, regret, and anger. I am totally amazed at the number of women who announce that they are celibate, yet the declaration is tinged with much frustration and negativity. I counseled a young man in Atlanta who was dating a celibate woman. Curtis is in his early thirties. He's a young, handsome, African American brother, and a talented artist. We've had numerous telephone-counseling sessions about his love life. He hopes to meet a nice woman with whom he can share his life. One day he met Tonya at the mall. She's in her late twenties, very beautiful, and she obviously had a mutual attraction to Curtis. She was from out of town, but they exchanged phone numbers and began a friendship.

After a month of long-distance calling, Curtis planned a trip to South Carolina to visit her for the weekend. He drove from Atlanta to South Carolina. He made reservations at a nearby hotel for himself. That evening he arrived at her home with a bouquet of lovely red roses. Before taking the flowers from him, she announced, "Don't think that because you brought me these flowers, we're having sex, 'cause I'm celibate! But you can stay in my guest room." Curtis was shocked at her outburst. Who was this woman, and what had she done with the Tonya on the phone? What had he done to warrant such an angry outburst? He kindly informed her that he already had a place to stay. He just wanted to take her to the movies and dinner, to get to know her a little better. After that, the weekend was enjoyable until he attended her church on Sunday. As soon as they entered the sanctuary, her grandmother, mother, aunts, cousins, and the rest of her family tree gathered around Curtis and began the sanctified version of twenty questions: "Are you saved, sanctified, Holy Ghost–filled, fire-baptized, on your way to heaven and enjoying the trip, and speaking in other tongues as Spirit gives you utterance?" Before he could respond, another branch of the tree asked, "Are you baptized in Jesus only? You ain't Catholic, are you?" Needless to say, after Curtis left Tonya's church, he drove back home to Atlanta and called me.

A state of celibacy is something people choose to enter into for a period of time to devote more of their energy and focus on the care and health of the soul, heart, and mind. Tonya was angry because she was celibate; it was not a condition she entered into with joy, but rather with regret and a heavy mandate from her religious tradition. We will talk more about celibacy later.

Some women do have a healthy sense of themselves and live

responsible lives in all areas—emotionally, spiritually, intellectually, and sexually. They are in a committed, monogamous relationship that may lead to marriage or may not, and they are okay with that. As spiritual women, they celebrate the gift of life that they have received from God, and they try to live life to the fullest every day, giving back to life in multiple ways. These sisters of spirit are in every walk of life. They are television talk-show hosts, news anchors, university professors, ministers, lawyers, hair stylists, actresses, musicians, presidents of corporations and foundations—all women who love God, love themselves, and love their neighbors. Women of spirit, who nurture their lives and try to walk in sanity and spiritual balance, are always mindful of the need to withdraw from others every now and then and dedicate a time of solitude and retreat with their Lord. This is the best condition for a time of celibacy. Dedicate a time of celibacy as a gift that you share with God in prayer, reflection, and meditation. Do not allow feelings of guilt, shame, and anger to drive you away from sexual intimacy with others. Rather, allow the call to celibacy to be a loving invitation to communion with God.

Could you relate to the stories of Tammy, Lisa, or Jennifer?
How so?

_____

_____

_____

_____

How do you feel about brothers who are on the sexual "down-
low"? What advice would you give a sister who is involved in such
a relationship and hoping to convert him?

_____

_____

_____

_____

Where are you on the spectrum from celibate to celebrate? Are you whole, satisfied, sane, and at peace? If not, what do you want to do to get to that place of joyful balance?

_____

_____

_____

_____

_____

How can I say "thank you" to God for my sexuality?

- By refusing to participate in soulless sex
- By choosing a season of celibacy to commune with God
- By realizing that lovemaking is a gift from God

CHAPTER SEVEN

Sexual Healing for the Church

He has told you, O mortal, what is good;
and what does the Lord require of you but to do justice,
and to love kindness, and to walk humbly with your God?

—MICAH 6:8

When the Black church is able to talk honestly about sex, teach about sex, and preach from the pulpit about issues related to sex—then we will begin to see powerful changes in the life of the black community. When the faith community is no longer sexually dysfunctional, then we will begin to see true abundant life in the lives of our women and men. But for that to happen, the church must find its voice and begin talking about issues that have been taboo for too long.

The Black church is *like* a dysfunctional family when it comes to the issue of sex. Similar to a clinically diagnosed dysfunctional family, the church has a sickness and everyone knows it, but no one says anything about it. Usually, one member of the family has a sickness: alcoholism, drug addiction, etc. The other members of the family do not acknowledge it or talk about it—it is the family secret. No one wants to bring disgrace to the family, so they keep quiet. The family secret affects everyone differently. In the typical family of dysfunction, there is a heroic child. This family over-achiever brings home all A's, wins the awards, excels academically or athletically. The child brings honor to the family, trying to re-deem the family name. Then there is the enabler of the family, usually the spouse of the person with the disease. He or she tries to please everyone, and will do whatever it takes to keep peace within the family, even to the point of self-sacrifice. Then there is the lost child, the black sheep. She seems self-destructive and is always in trouble. She never seems to accomplish anything of great worth. She usually does not want to have anything to do with the family of origin and withdraws. No one blames her; they understand that she missed out on a happy childhood because of the family secret.

The problem with this type of family situation is that no one will be healed until the person with the disease is healed. And the person with the disease will never be healed until someone who truly cares about his health, wholeness, and well-being confronts him in truth and love about his illness. Usually, whoever does this will not be liked by any member of the family or by the person with the illness. Everyone is too invested in keeping the family se-cret. For the person with the sickness to get help, everyone must be involved. All the family members have gotten used to their broken lives. They have become accustomed to walking with a limp. They have adjusted their bodies to walk with their burden, and they are convinced that it is not as heavy as they originally thought—they have long forgotten about trying to lay the bur-den down. To do so makes them now feel naked and exposed.

Unfortunately, when one member of a family has a sickness, everyone suffers with symptoms.

When I am invited to preach on Women's Day, I must admit that in some churches I am very aware there is sickness present. Yes, it is Women's Day, the women are in their white, the choir is full of sisters singing the praises of God. The pulpit is full of women, some clergy and some laity, all leading worship in one manner or another. Spiritually, it is a high and festive time. Often, the pastor (usually male) sits in the front row with the other male clergy or with the deacons. On a few occasions, the pastor has sat in the pulpit, which is appropriate since he is the pastor, but once in a while the pastor does not grant me the "preacher's chair," which is rude by anyone's standards, especially the unwritten but clearly understood code of conduct for clergy. However, this is not what disturbs me the most. I cannot avoid realizing that on the following Sunday, the women clergy and laity who lead the worship today will once again be lost in the crowd. The deaconess who offers the morning prayer and stands at the altar while I "open the doors of the church" will not stand there again until another fifty-two Sundays have passed. There is a sickness in the Black church, and it is the sometimes subsiding, but never dying, sexism.

Women have been told we should be grateful that we are granted a Women's Day, that women are allowed in the pulpit, that the woman preacher can preach from the pulpit rather than from the floor. We should not complain or even speak of any dissatisfaction. This reminds me of white America during segregation, telling us that we should be thankful for what they have afforded us, and that coloreds need to remember their place.

I remember becoming acutely aware of this sickness in the Black church when I was wrestling with my call to the ministry. I was a member of a very loving and warm Baptist church. The pastor was a great preacher and an excellent teacher. In April 1976, when I told him that I'd been called to preach, his reply was, "Susan, I knew that when you joined here; it's written all over you." I shadowed him when he visited the sick, preached away at revivals. Later, when he had to be gone, he asked me to teach his Bible class. I preached my initial sermon in September of that same year, and was licensed into the ministry. At that time there were five other associate ministers at the church—one woman and four men. Every Sunday, the women sat in the congregation and the men sat with the pastor in the pulpit. However, twice a year we were allowed in the pulpit—Women's Day and Missionary Sunday. The other woman minister was the chair of the missionaries, and she always preached on Missionary Sunday. As in most churches, the associates don't get to preach often unless it's at the eight A.M. service, but for the sisters it was even less frequent. I remember asking to preach the three A.M. Halloween service. I was joking, but there often is much truth in a joke.

The major realization came when I entered Wesley Theological Seminary in the fall of 1978, and a few of the male officers of the church talked with me about how it was not necessary for me to go to seminary. I was told that the Holy Ghost would teach me what I needed to know. They affirmed their love and support for me and my ministry, but stated that I did not have to become ordained. I discovered that the Baptist Minister's Conference of Washington, D.C., and Vicinity would not ordain a woman and that any church that did so was excommunicated from the conference. My pastor was an active member of this group. I knew that if I finished seminary, I would want to pastor a church or do ministry and would need to be ordained. Seeking to do so would put my pastor in political hot water. I could tell from our conversations that he was beginning to feel differently about women in pastoral ministry because he mentored me and could not deny the gifts and graces of God present in my life.

So I dropped out of seminary after one semester. One Sunday afternoon during Holy Communion service, I saw in a new way something very ordinary about our worship service, and for the first time it provided an extraordinary jolt to my consciousness. After the pastor preached, he and the men would leave the pulpit and offer the right hand of fellowship to the new members, and the women clergy in the congregation would join them in this ritual of love. After shaking the new members' hands, the men would sit behind the communion table, and the women clergy would return to our seats in the congregation. By this time there were ten associate ministers—six men and four women. Of the six men, three were my students in Bible study. One of the men was recently licensed, nineteen years old, and a first-semester student in college. The only differences between the two of us was that I was five years older, had more theological training, and did not have a penis.

I knew no matter what anyone else said, I had to be true to what God had placed in my spirit. I entered Howard University Divinity School in the fall of 1979. As in any graduate school, whether medical, law, or business, as a seminarian I had to complete an internship. Because I wanted to intern for a church where I could fully exercise my gifts for my calling every Sunday, not just one Sunday out of fifty-two, I left the church of my heart and went where I could serve without restrictions.

Sexism is the Black church's sickness; it is the family secret. We know it exists, but no one says anything. Some women may get mad about it, but then we are granted a women's ministry or fellowship and we get quiet for a while. Most ministers confronted with the issue of sexism will readily point to one or two women on their trustee board, or women licensed and sitting in the pulpit, but the very fact that we as a people can still easily count who we have in what places is painful. The articles in *Jet* and *Ebony* announce with celebration, "The African Methodist Episcopal Church elects the first woman Bishop, Dr. Vashti McKenzie." I was ecstatic when I heard the news. Vashti is a friend and beloved sister, but what took so long, brothers? I applaud the pastors who do treat the male and female clergy of their churches with equality, but these pastors are too few. For some of my own friends I've helped prepare a church budget for the trustee board meeting, or counseled them on how to transition from their secular jobs to become full-time pastors, yet I've never graced their pulpits. These are men who cannot deny the gift of God within their sisters, but they have no confidence in them simply because they are women. I understand not having an associate, whether male or female, perform a certain task because of lack of experience, but when it is obvious that a woman is experienced and capable and she still is not allowed to enter certain areas of pastoral duties, then I would ask for a reality check; more often than not, the diagnosis will still be sexism.

There is an unexpressed power within spiritual women. For a woman of spirit to be unlimited in her creativity and self-expression can be misinterpreted and threatening to some men. Women of spirit can preach, teach, pastor, chair the joint boards, serve on the city council, sit in Congress, fly into space, dive to the ocean's floor, climb the mountain's heights, cook, clean, conceive a life in our wombs, nurture it within for nine months, and birth into the world a child who may be the Savior of the world—that's powerful! But the gift that men often overlook is that women of spirit desire to be trusted and loved by our brothers, in order that we may do the will of God in this world together. In 1888, a black women's advocate, Ellen Watkins Harper, speaking at a gathering, said, "Great evils stare us in the face that need to be throttled by the combined power of an upright manhood and an enlightened womanhood; and I know that no nation can gain its full measure of enlightenment and happiness if one half of it is free and the other half is fettered. China compressed the feet of her women and thereby retarded the steps of her men. No nation can be strong when one half of its people are fettered, and the other half is free."

If a man has a heart attack and is rushed to the emergency room, do you think he would care if the cardiologist is a man or a woman? I don't think so; he should care only that the doctor is qualified and skilled enough to save his life. It will take the men and women of God, working as colleagues and partners, to deliver our families and communities from the vicissitudes of life that oppress us still. This may sound harsh, but the truth of the matter is, if you don't want women to preach, pastor, counsel, or teach, then don't preach, pastor, counsel, or teach them. If you will not ordain women into the ministry, then stop baptizing them. No man has power over the movement of the Spirit of God. Once the liberating Gospel of Jesus Christ is preached and the Word is planted in a sister's heart, there are no limits to what God's Spirit will direct her to do. So if you never let a woman experience the love of God, then maybe she won't preach, prophesy, or proclaim it. But I'm afraid you're too late.

Our black communities are in desperate need of every available loving heart and hand to work for the deliverance of our children and their families. While the church is silent, too many people are becoming infected with HIV/AIDS. While the church is silent, women are suffering sexual and physical abuse. While the church is silent, children are sexually molested. While the church is silent, teenagers are becoming parents too soon.

The Black church has always been the beacon of hope in the black community. The Black church has historically been the one place that colored, Negro, black, African American people have owned and operated. When we were slaves, our foreparents found solace as they gathered at the river and around campfires to pray and hear a Word from the Lord. During the days of Jim Crow, night riders, KKK, and lynchings, it was the Black church and the black preacher who offered help and hope to our families. Before we had federal government programs to aid struggling families, it was the church that offered education, job training, food, and shelter through the missionary department and benevolent societies. Whenever an injustice occurred, we fought it. Whenever a people were oppressed, we were there, marching, protesting, shouting, preaching, praying, proclaiming, giving, exhorting, crying, working. We have stared down sickness, poverty, unemployment, racism, water hoses, and vicious dogs; now our communities are threatened by something that has no cure—HIV/AIDS. The only weapon we have is educating people to change their behavior. Yet the loudest, most influential voice in the history of Africans in America sits in the pulpit and pews of our churches silent on Sunday.

This is not like us. We are a compassionate people. We know how it feels to be threatened, abandoned, left behind, oppressed, isolated, misunderstood, ostracized, ridiculed, spat upon, and unfairly judged based on an outward label, rather than an inner love. This is not a time for us to be silent!

African Americans account for 13 percent of the U.S. population. Yet they account for nearly 50 percent of AIDS cases. By the year 2005, that figure is expected to rise to 60 percent. Currently,

1 in 50 black men is HIV positive, and 1 in 160 black women is positive. Black senior citizens represent more than 50 percent of HIV cases among persons over age fifty-five.

Churches can have ministries that educate our community about HIV/AIDS, teen pregnancy prevention, domestic violence, sexual abuse, rape, birth control, and many other critical issues related to sex. But when this suggestion is made, issues arise that serve to paralyze the successful implementation of such educational programs and critically needed ministries.

The primary hurdle that arises around the initiation of any HIV/AIDS ministry in our churches is the issue of homosexuality. I'm not going to rehash all the arguments because you know them already and have probably participated in a debate about homosexuality in the church, but let me say this: While we in the church spend so much precious time and energy arguing about where the viruses came from, whether this is God's judgment upon gay people, whether it was a government conspiracy that created the virus in a laboratory, or any of the hundreds of other inane discussions, millions of people are becoming infected and dying! We are wasting time!

No matter what the issues are in our society, in our neighborhoods, and in our faith communities, there is only *one* thing required of God's people: "To do justice, and to love kindness, and to walk humbly with your God" (Micah 6:8). That's it! The church's role is not to be the seek-and-destroy squad or to play the blame game. Of all the organizations, agencies, and groups in our communities, the church's role is to do whatever is necessary to create and promote healing in the lives of people. We are to be loving and forgiving.

Some heterosexual men and women live and treat one another in ways that are an abomination, but we don't talk about that.

Some women and children suffer actions that are not loving or life-nurturing as abominable things are done to them in homes across America every day, but we don't talk about that. Some men and women who use sex to manipulate others to their will or to enforce their selfish desires perform abominable acts every day, but we don't talk about that. But when we find a woman loving another woman, or learn of two women who love each other and want to buy a house in our community, we cry "Abomination!" and strategize to find ways to keep them outside of our neighborhood.

Sarah is a thirty-two-year-old woman who has dedicated her life to helping single mothers in Georgia find work and support for themselves and their children. Hundreds of women who have been abandoned by their men must find work that pays them a livable wage, so they can afford child care, health insurance, food, clothing, and housing. These are the mothers whom Sarah has worked with for the past ten years, moving them from welfare to work and beyond. She has successfully lobbied the state legislature and governor's office for greater benefits and a higher quality of life for hundreds of women in Georgia. She has received numerous awards for her life's work. Sarah is a lesbian. She has been in a committed, monogamous relationship with her companion for fifteen years.

In Luke 10:25–37, we find this poignant lesson:

> Just then a lawyer stood up to test Jesus. "Teacher," he said, "what must I do to inherit eternal life?" He said to him, "What is written in the law? What do you read there?" He answered, "You shall love the Lord your God with all your heart, and with all your soul, and with all your strength, and with all your mind; and your neighbor

as yourself." And he said to him, "You have given the right answer; do this, and you will live." But wanting to justify himself, he asked Jesus, "And who is my neighbor?" Jesus replied, "A man was going down from Jerusalem to Jericho, and fell into the hands of robbers, who stripped him, beat him, and went away, leaving him half dead. Now by chance a priest was going down that road; and when he saw him, he passed by on the other side. So likewise a Levite, when he came to the place and saw him, he passed by on the other side. But a Samaritan while traveling came near him; and when he saw him, he was moved with pity. He went to him and bandaged his wounds, having poured oil and wine on them. Then he put him on his own animal, brought him to an inn, and took care of him. The next day he took out two denarii, gave them to the innkeeper, and said, 'Take care of him; and when I come back, I will repay you whatever more you spend.' Which of these three, do you think, was a neighbor to the man who fell into the hands of the robbers?" He said, "The one who showed him mercy." Jesus said to him, "Go and do likewise."

So when I answer the question, Who in my life has been Christlike or like the good Samaritan, the individual I think of is not always a heterosexual person. When I was away from home, sick, and in the hospital, and I needed someone to come stay with me and help nurse me back to health, who came without any excuses or reservations? A bisexual man. When I could not pay my mortgage because I was recently unemployed and my former church had voted not to grant me severance pay, who came and lived in my home and paid half the mortgage, bought food, cooked, and cleaned my home until I was able to do for myself? Two of my friends—a lesbian couple—who have been in a committed monogamous relationship for several years.

Jesus said:

> Then the king will say to those at his right hand, "Come, you that are blessed by my Father, inherit the kingdom prepared for you from the foundation of the world; for I was hungry and you gave me food, I was thirsty and you gave me something to drink, I was a stranger and you welcomed me, I was naked and you gave me clothing, I was sick and you took care of me, I was in prison and you visited me." Then the righteous will answer him, "Lord, when was it that we saw you hungry and gave you food, or thirsty and gave you something to drink? And when was it that we saw you a stranger and welcomed you, or naked and gave you clothing? And when was it that we saw you sick or in prison and visited you?" And the king will answer them, "Truly I tell you, just as you did it to one of the least of these who are members of my family, you did it to me" (Matthew 25:34–40).

Teen pregnancy among black females aged fifteen to nineteen fell 21 percent last year. However, a 13 percent increase is predicted by 2005, according to the U.S. Centers for Disease Control and Prevention.

The church in its role as educator cannot teach classes on self-esteem only to teenage girls; it must reach out to adult women as well. A seminar on Becoming Whole Through Self-Love would be a powerful witness of the greatest commandment—"You shall love the Lord your God with all your heart, and with all your soul, and with all your strength, and with all your mind; and your neighbor *as yourself*" (Luke 10:17). Dr. Kelly Brown Douglas, womanist theologian and author of *Sexuality and the Black Church*, writes, "A new Black perspective on sexuality must begin with those who constitute over 70 percent of Black church congregations, Black women. When Black women are able to affirm themselves and come to a healthy sense of their own sexuality, patterns of relationships are transformed for the entire Black community."

The Black church can begin to talk about sex and related topics from a new perspective. There are numerous complex issues involved in black life, and most churches have people in the pews who can offer their skills in a shared ministry with the clergy. We have excelled in implementing ministries like day care, senior citizens' housing, meals on wheels, credit unions, and much more. Now, let us go on to the greater things that we can accomplish together, like a crisis referral service for victims of domestic violence, rape, sexual abuse, incest, etc. (See the "Resources" section at the end of this book.)

If Jesus were pastoring a church today, what kind of ministries would there be at His church? What do you think the role of women would be?

_____

_____

_____

_____

Have you noticed symptoms of sexism in your church? How do you feel about it, and what can you do to begin to change it?

_____

_____

_____

_____

Do you know any people in your family or circle of friends living with HIV/AIDS? Would your church be open and affirming of them?

_____

_____

_____

_____

Are you willing to become a "sex-talker"? How would you start the conversation in your church?

_____

_____

_____

_____

Chapter Eight

A New Sexual Ethic for the Spiritual Woman

Do not remember the former things, or consider the things of old. I am
about to do a new thing; now it springs forth; do you not perceive it?

—ISAIAH 43:18–19

We've taken an honest look at ourselves and our ideas about sex.
We've reflected upon our first lessons about sex. We've examined
the teachings of the Bible in relation to sex. We've quoted and
memorized words of inspiration. We've affirmed ourselves, written
prayers, and recorded things in our journals that we didn't even
know existed in our hearts. We have reclaimed our bodies with
positive self-images. We now know that we can love God and sex,
too. We've discovered a new freedom about sex. What now? Do
we run out the gate, bucking like wild animals in heat? No, not
at all.

I thought this would be the part in the book where I give
you the Seven Steps to Sexual and Spiritual Union, or the Ten

Commandments of Sex. But none of these approaches would be possible because I do not see this new ethic as something that pertains only to sexual ethics. I see this as a whole new paradigm of how we can live every aspect of our lives as women of spirit. I don't just desire women to change their thinking about their sexual principles with just a few prayers, meditations, and affirmations, I want women to begin looking at their entire lives from a new place—within their own spirit and heart. Spiritual women, as a part of their ever growing relationship with God, can enter into a covenant with God, the end result of their spiritual transformation to a higher knowledge of their own spirit and a deeper, more personal way to walk with the Lord. This new ethic is firmly rooted in what Jesus called "the greatest commandment."

> And one of them, a lawyer, asked him a question to test him. "Teacher, which commandment in the law is the greatest?" He said to him, " 'You shall love the Lord your God with all your heart, and with all your soul, and with all your mind.' This is the greatest and first commandment. And a second is like it: 'You shall love your neighbor as yourself.' On these two commandments hang all the law and the prophets." (Matthew 22:35–39)

This should be the spiritual foundation for all of our lives, regardless of religious beliefs, culture, or creed. As people of faith and spirit, we should love God first and foremost, love ourselves, and love our neighbors. Wherever we are, God is. There is nothing we can do and nowhere we can go where God is not present. In theological terms, God is omnipresent—fully everywhere at the same time. There is no aspect of our lives in which God is not with us. God is present with us in our successes and failures, in our pain and in our passion. There is no duality in God; therefore, there ought not to be any duality in the children of God. God is with us when we experience spiritual rapture and sexual ecstasy. Women of spirit can expand their lives, turn their personal world right side up, and live a more abundant life by just being honest and real about who they are, what they want, and how willing they are to know God and themselves on a deeper level.

Women are intelligent. Every day in America, a woman makes an important decision as a doctor, senator, corporate executive, mayor, mother, publisher, teacher, pharmacist, chef, engineer, or scientist. The intelligent woman who casts a vote on the floor of the Senate this morning is the same woman who decides to make love to her companion that night. She does not leave her intelligence in the Senate chamber, then transform into a senseless, hedonistic woman at home. A spiritual woman, who has a healthy love of self and an abiding relationship with God, is able to be guided by Spirit in every aspect of her life, but it takes a spiritual transformation to arrive at this new paradigm.

I'm not going to tell you what you should do. I want to encourage *you* to use the mind that God gave you, and the Holy Spirit that guides your life, to begin living a life that nurtures you, fulfills you, empowers you, and liberates you to be the self-confident woman of God that you were created to be. In the past, you have been guided by the religious teachings of your church, your parents, and the traditions of your culture. These have all served you well and have brought you to this present moment. But there comes a time when we all should examine who we are and what we believe and ask, Is this mine or someone else's?

It is not enough for you to live out the religious rituals of your mother or father. You must have a spiritual walk that is your own. You must have a relationship with God that is open, clear, honest, and individual. When you stand before God and no one else is around, talk with Him as you would your most intimate friends. Call God by whatever name feels most personal to you: Lord, Jesus, God, Heavenly Father, Holy One, Spirit Divine, Divine Presence, Father/Mother God, Savior, Yahweh, Allah, Abba, and so forth. This is between you and your Creator. This is personal and powerful. For when all is said and done, when you reach the end of your life, it's just going to be you and your God.

Many of you know the words of the scripture chapter and verse. If I begin a verse, you very likely can finish it. "For the one who is in you is greater than the one who is in the world" (I John 4:4). "No weapon that is fashioned against you shall prosper" (Isaiah 54:17). "No one has greater love than this, to lay down one's life for one's friends" (John 15:13). "For by grace you have been saved through faith, and this is not your own doing; it is the gift of God" (Ephesians 2:8). "For God so loved the world that he gave his only Son, so that everyone who believes in him may not perish but may have eternal life" (John 3:16). A great number of you were saying these scriptures right along with me. Some of you may not know them verbatim, but you were familiar with them.

The Holy Bible is a collection of sixty-six individual books. The Greek word *biblios* means little books. The Hebrew Bible, what Christians call the Old Testament, contains the writings about a people and their history with God. The New Testament contains the four Gospels that give a narrative account of the life and ministry of Jesus Christ. The rest of the New Testament contains letters that were written to members of this new religious sect called Christianity. The pastors and religious leaders of this group would write to the churches to give instruction, inspiration, correction, and edification. Most of the letters were written by a very popular and industrious pastor and teacher, Paul of Tarsus. Paul's popularity with the early churches reminds me of the popularity of Dr. Martin Luther King Jr. during the civil rights movement.

African Americans were being oppressed in their country, treated like second-class citizens, but they believed that their God had not forsaken them and would raise up someone to lead them to a better life. Dr. King was an accidental leader of his people, just as Paul was. Dr. King was a new pastor in Montgomery, Alabama. He did not accept the pastorate there to lead any type of movement, he just wanted to be a good pastor to his people. Paul, a member of the Pharisees, hated Christians and did everything within his power to destroy them. Then one day, God stepped into Martin's history, just as He had stepped into Paul's history.

Martin was chosen by his people to champion the cause of the oppressed. Paul became the victor of a people he once oppressed— the Christians. Martin was often misunderstood, beaten, hosed down in the streets, attacked by dogs, and jailed for what he accomplished on behalf of God's people. Paul was beaten, shipwrecked, left for dead, stoned, lashed, and jailed for what he accomplished on behalf of God's people. Paul wrote letters from his jail cell to encourage his people. He wrote as a first-century Jewish man. One who was raised on the Law of Moses but was learning to lean on the love and grace of Jesus. Martin wrote letters from his jail cell as well. There were religious leaders who did not think he should try to change the traditions and lifestyles of the people in the South. These clergy tried to persuade him to stop his agitation, to stop his fight for the freedom of his people. They tried to point out the dangers that existed if he kept moving in this new direction. But Martin wrote the clergy a letter from his Birmingham jail, answering their demands that he should wait.

His letters have been published in a book titled *Why We Can't Wait*. Some of the apostle Paul's letters were included in the canon of the Bible.

These two were God-anointed men who pastored a nation of people and provided spiritual guidance. One must be able to read their letters and writings to glean the eternal truths of the universe of good and evil, justice and injustice, love and hate. Though their writings were influenced by their own traditions and the customs of their time, that does not take away the great value of the eternal truths inherent in their inspired words.

Thomas Jefferson was one of the founding fathers of this nation who crafted the Declaration of Independence. He wrote, "We hold these truths to be self-evident, that all men are created equal, that they are endowed by their Creator with certain unalienable Rights, that among these are Life, Liberty and the pursuit of Happiness." But this same man owned slaves. Like Paul, he was a man of great character and power, whose writings and work changed the very course of history. But one has to be able to look upon these men and separate their good works from their beliefs and practices as men of their times.

Albert Einstein said, "We cannot solve problems we have created with the same thinking that created them." In other words, we are unable to solve the problems we have created with the same theologizing and church practices that have created them. Dr. Cornel West, speaking at the Balm in Gilead's AIDS and the Black Church conference, said, "Just have enough courage to be yourself, you see, because the most difficult thing for a human being, especially a Black person, is to be themselves. But keep in mind that the most dangerous person in America is a self-loving, self-respecting Black person. . . . And the question is, are you going to allow the Gospel to free you enough, do you trust Jesus enough, are you willing to make the leap of faith and step out on nothing and land on something?"

What both men were asking are important questions for people who say they believe in a God who "is able to accomplish abundantly far more than all we can ask or imagine" (Ephesians 3:20). Many people are afraid of doing new things or accepting an alternative way of living. We are creatures of habit and don't like to change. For every new thing that comes up related to the spiritual life, someone will ask the question, What does the Bible say about it? Well, to be honest, the Bible does not speak directly to many things in life. This does not mean that the Bible is irrelevant to our lives today. The Bible is full of the stories of men and women of faith that point to the love of God for God's people. But, unfortunately, some have taken the instructions that are particular to that culture and time as commandments of God.

A New Sexual Ethic of Honesty

Our new sexual ethic is based on believing that we have the freedom to choose how we express ourselves sexually. We learn to apply lessons gleaned from past relationships. As spiritual women, we know that "whatsoever we sow, that shall we reap." We cannot afford to live our lives carelessly. Every aspect of life needs forethought and planning. No endeavor should be undertaken without an honest conversation with our highest self, asking, Is this what I want? Is this right for me?

In thousands of Baptist churches around the world, once a month Holy Communion is celebrated. Before partaking of the bread and cup, members of the congregation read the church covenant in unison—that is, until they get to one particular part where everyone seems to get something stuck in their throats and begin to cough. "Having been led as we believe, by the Spirit of God to receive the Lord Jesus Christ . . . we do now in the presence of God, angels, and this assembly, most solemnly and joyfully enter into covenant with one another, as one body in Christ . . . we promise to abstain from the sale (coughing) and use of intoxicating drink as a beverage." Though everyone reads this covenant, many drink alcoholic beverages. A glass of white Zinfandel at a business reception is commonplace for many. Enjoying a cold one at a football game or a cookout with family is a weekly occurrence. Many Christians choose to enjoy alcoholic beverages as a part of their lifestyle, but they do not want anyone outside of their inner circle to know, thereby exposing themselves to the judgment and scrutiny of others.

When I was a new World Mission Support field counselor for the American Baptist Churches USA, a group of us were at the headquarters in Valley Forge, Pennsylvania, for orientation. After a long day of work, we all went to dinner. We were Baptist ministers—male and female, black, Latino, and white, and from various parts of the country. The waiter came to our table and asked, "May I start you off with a cocktail?" A white minister from Georgia spoke up as if insulted by the question, "Sir, we are Baptist ministers! We do not drink alcoholic beverages [pause] with each other."

As people of faith and spirit, there are many things that we will not *do* with each other that we may do when alone or with another, more intimate group of friends. It is unfortunate that we feel the need to live such a dual life because of what others may say or how others may judge us. But to be healthy, whole, sane women of God, we must be honest about our love for God and our desire for companionship that includes sexual intimacy.

I have preached and conducted women's retreats all across this country, and in every one there is the seminar after the seminar. In the evening after the day's workshops have ended, a group of women will invariably come to my room or will join me for dinner to talk about sex. These are wonderful, spiritual women who are dedicated and committed to their work in the church. Many of them were raised in the church. Some of them have positions of leadership in the church—clergy, deaconesses, trustees, Sunday school teachers, choir members, ushers, etc. They are not sluts, ho's, bitches, or freaks, but sex is an important part of their relationships with their boyfriends and companions.

Some of these women are single and looking to marry. Others who are divorced or widowed are not looking for another husband, but they have a healthy libido and don't want to stop being sexually active. Still others don't plan on ever marrying, but they want sexual intimacy in their lives. The jist of the conversation is to understand how they can have such feelings of love, attraction, and affection for someone while being told by the church that sharing this feeling through the act of making love is a sin. It comes down to one's ethics—what are your standards for your own sex life?

Ethics or morals are always an issue when contemplating sex. Ethical standards have traditionally brought up the question of what is right and wrong, as if everything were black and white, with no gray areas. For some, morals serve as a hindrance to sex, as if it is the role of morals to keep sex under control, restricted, or limited in its full expression. The sex lives of many would improve if they were willing to come to terms with guilt and shame that they may have associated with sex, and find a sexual ethic with which they can peacefully live—one based upon truth.

In order to have a compassionate, joyful, and mature morality, you must first have an honest heart-to-heart talk with yourself and your God. Many have a dried-up morality that serves to hinder sexual pleasure rather than to remind and guide the responsibilities of sexual expression. Your principles of morality should be created out of personal reflection and honest conversation with self first, and a fiercely honest relationship with God. You can lie to other people, and you can lie to yourself for a little while, but you cannot lie to God. Be honest about your sexual feelings and beliefs. No one else lives in your body but you, and no one has to stand before God but you alone.

Some people are very outspoken about their moral standards in regard to sex. The very fact that they protest so much is a dead giveaway that they, themselves, are struggling with a sexual dilemma. Sometimes the struggle they have is like a compulsion to flee from the very thing to which they are so strongly drawn. I think of one popular televangelist who used to preach so much against the lust of the flesh, only to be discovered several months later having sex with prostitutes in motels. Former FBI director J. Edgar Hoover was obsessed with taping and gathering information about the sexual liaisons of various people in public life, while he was a cross-dresser. A wise person once said, "People in glass houses should not throw stones."

I am all for people having moral standards to live by and hold firmly to, if they truly *believe* in those standards. But if you are struggling to live by someone else's ethics, then you need to reexamine them carefully to see if you can accept them as yours. So many people are trying to live by someone else's standards. Ethics are like a custom-made suit; if they weren't tailor-made for you, their fit will always be uncomfortable, and you will eventually discard them.

Most people do not take the time to question why they

believe what they believe or do what they do; they behave as they do because everyone else is doing the same or because someone told them it was the right action to take. Well, that's fine at first, but later on you should consider it for yourself. I moved into my first apartment when I was twenty-five. I bought all the stuff I'd need to furnish my home and make it livable. From that day to this, wherever I've lived there is always a wooden rolling pin and wax paper in the kitchen drawer. I do not make pie crust from scratch, but I have a rolling pin and wax paper because my mother always had them in her kitchen. And if my mother did it, then I would do it without a second thought.

One day, I began to rethink doing everything my mother told me. When I was a child, my mother was like God to me. Everything she said to do, I did without much fuss or question, because she was the mother and I was the child. It never occurred to me that I should think for myself about some things. Then one day I saw Momma in a different light. One winter, after a night of snow and ice, someone broke into Momma's Oldsmobile Cutlass Supreme. He was unsuccessful in stealing it; someone frightened him away. The next day, Momma asked James (my husband at the time) and a family friend to go have a car alarm installed. That evening, they took Momma outside to show her how to arm and disarm the car. When she returned, I noticed she had the owner's manual in her hand (it usually stayed in the glove compartment). Momma put the book in the bureau's top drawer and proclaimed, "There, the next time if anyone tries to steal the car, they won't know how to drive it off!" Well, after we got up off the floor with tears in our eyes, I said, "Momma, a car thief doesn't need the owner's manual to steal the car." I knew then and there that I needed to do a lot more thinking for myself.

Spiritual women who are ready to live more complete, balanced, wholesome lives can achieve sexual and spiritual union through honesty about themselves and a closer relationship with God. To be sexually aroused and then try to deny our body's natural expression is to deny the very essence of who God created us to be—sexual beings, with spirit, mind, heart, and soul. But as spiritual people, our lives should show moderation and balance in all we do. This is not easy, and these goals are not achieved overnight, but every journey begins with a first step.

God's Spirit residing within our hearts gives us little nudges about choices we make, but a great deal of the time we ignore Spirit. I believe that a woman's intuition is an expression of Spirit in our lives. Intuition is like the wisdom of Spirit speaking to us. All of us have been told to "listen to your inner voice, trust your instincts." I automatically picture Luke Skywalker being mentored by Yoda in *Star Wars*. Luke would try to rely solely upon his five senses and skill, but Yoda taught him to focus on the Force and guidance from within. This is what we call walking by faith, not by sight. As spiritual men and women, we have neglected nurturing the attributes and characteristics of Spirit in our lives. The greatest manifestation of the Divine Presence is from within.

This is the importance of the disciplines of the Spirit in our lives—contemplative prayer, meditation, fasting, solitude, worship, etc. Richard J. Foster, in his book *Celebration of Discipline: The Path to Spiritual Growth*, says that if we believe that we live in a universe created by the infinite-personal God "who delights in our communion with him, you will see meditation as communication between the Lover and the beloved." For far too long we have neglected our own spiritual growth, not knowing that the balance and sanity we so long for in life can only be borne upon the wings of the Spirit.

The Russian mystic Theophan the Recluse says, "To pray is to descend with the mind into the heart, and there to stand before the face of the Lord, ever-present, all seeing, within you." To step outside of your usual mundane religious rituals and go deeper into the presence of God through an inward journey of Spirit will usher you into the presence of God in a new and powerful way. It is here, at this level of spiritual strength and intimacy, that the lines of demarcation between spirituality and sexuality begin to dissolve. When you stand naked before the presence of God in a deeper relationship as lover and beloved, you will discover the sacredness of your own sexuality and the sensuousness of your spirit. None of this takes away from the religious teachings of your childhood; it transforms your spiritual understanding to a new dimension of God consciousness.

Whether in church, mosque, or temple, women of spirit need to begin having open and honest conversations about living an unfettered life in the presence of God's Spirit. There are thousands of women who spend hundreds of dollars flying across the country to attend yet another conference on women and spirit. These women have a wonderful time in praise and worship, but they come back home just as bound up, acknowledging feeling the presence of Spirit in their lives, and yet guilt-ridden about their desire to be fully expressive in relationship with their companions.

It is time for us to look critically at the religious beliefs we have worn for years, and at how our day-to-day practices may differ from the biblical principles that we accept. Many may not agree that this kind of dichotomy is possible or desirable. Periodically, however, we should examine ourselves to see what we believe and how that relates to our personal walk with the Lord. Some who are trying to walk in someone else's shoes are walking with a limp.

SEX WITH THAT ONE SPECIAL SOMEONE

In some cultures it is said that to have sex with someone is to know the person in a deep way, and to have sex for the first time is to know life in a way that is entirely new and transforming. Sex is a kind of gnosis, or holy knowing. In Genesis, after Adam and Eve were created, the Bible says, "[Adam] *knew* his wife Eve, and she conceived and bore Cain" (Genesis 4:1). This *knowing* creates a bond between the partners. Many try to keep sex as something purely physical so they do not have to deal with the feelings and repercussions attached with the sexual act. The attempt to have sex without implications may backfire, and through a meaningless sexual fling we may find ourselves in the biggest emotional mess of our lives.

In July 2001, David Satcher, the U.S. Surgeon General, announced the Surgeon General's Call to Action to Promote Sexual Health and Responsible Sexual Behavior. In his call to action, Dr. Satcher stressed the importance of individuals being in committed, monogamous sexual relationships. Well, you would have thought he called for the death of every firstborn child. He was condemned by the conservative religious right for promoting sex outside of marriage. The reality is, millions of people are sexually active with multiple partners, and at risk for infection. Therefore, bedside advice of the nation's personal physician is to "love thy neighbor, not thy neighborhood!"

A SEASON OF CELIBACY

For many, celibacy is a preferred choice. For the purpose of our discussion, celibacy is making the decision to abstain from sexual intercourse when there is no healthy, loving, monogamous, committed relationship present in our life. Being involved in a sexual relationship without monogamy or commitment is referred to as recreational sex.

Recreational or casual sex is dangerous for many reasons. First, casual sex is unhealthy. With the pandemic of HIV/AIDS and other sexually transmitted diseases, a woman is playing the odds with her life when she is casual about sexual partners and practices. Second, casual sex may be detrimental to your heart. Some women who seek intimacy from a man will settle for sex instead of love—they often get confused because both feel good. How many times can you fall in and out of love with a man, not to mention in and out of bed, before your heart suffers a lack-of-love attack?

It's the easiest thing in the world to have sex with a man; the real challenge is to have a relationship with a man based on friendship, respect, and affection. Don't get me wrong, I know that the physical attraction plays a major part, but usually that's what gets folks into trouble—they are hormone directed rather than heart directed. Your hormones will tell you, "You need to get some of that now," but your heart is saying, "Let's get to know him better first." I know, you're thinking, Ain't no man going to delay sex in order to get to know me first, there's too many women out there who will give him what he wants now. Well, if that is the case, then you have to ask yourself the hard, honest questions: Is this what I want? Do I feel respected and loved by him?

No man is going to respect and love you until you respect and love yourself first. If you are desperate and will do anything to hold on to a man, he knows it. If you are insecure and clingy, he knows it. If you are obsessive and plan your entire day around his phone call, his e-mail, or the slightest bit of attention from him, he knows he has you, and the excitement of the chase is gone. There is no mystique, no challenge, nothing to look forward to. I'm not saying play hard to get or any of those games that girls play. But, as a woman of spirit, I am saying to nurture and love yourself in such a way that others will notice your confidence, self-love, and calm assurance, and they will want to know you and love you, too.

No one can use you without your permission. Many women are so glad to have a man in their lives and in their beds that they lower their standards for a mate or companion. I remember when we were young girls in high school or college, we'd sit around and daydream about our husbands and what characteristics and traits we desired in our perfect love. Our descriptions went something like this: "He must be tall with broad shoulders. I want a man with a wonderful personality who is easy to get along with. Someone very successful in his business. He owns his own home, and drives an expensive car. He's not stingy and does not mind lavishing me with gifts."

Now, years later, the only requirement some women have for a companion is that he be male and in good health. If he's unemployed, we'll pay his bills and give him money. If he's without transportation, we'll let him drive our car until we can buy him one. If he doesn't buy us gifts for our birthday or holidays, we make up excuses to our family and friends that he's a member of a religious group that doesn't believe in that sort of thing. We find ourselves settling for whatever comes along, rather than choosing a companion who is worthy of us. We are Queens and the daughters of a living God—we deserve the *best*. So, as Iyanla says, *In the Meantime,* we continue to love ourselves and cherish our friends and work on what I like to call Project Me!

Project Me is based upon the greatest commandment, to love God, love self, and love your neighbor. Far too many women are loving the neighborhood and not paying attention to themselves.

Some women are so *otherly* directed that they neglect their own needs. Most women live their lives as the pivotal person for their children, their husband, their boss, their club, their church organizations. At the end of the day, there is no love left for self. This has to change, beginning *today*.

To begin Project Me, start by being committed to developing a relationship with yourself. We get so committed to other relationships that we only get around to our needs eventually, which often translates into never. When you begin to carve out time for yourself each day, you will be surprised to discover who you really are. You may find out that you are your favorite person and will want to spend more time with you!

Start respecting and cherishing yourself. Learn how to say no to others in order to say yes to yourself sometimes. This is not being selfish, this is being self-loving. The commandment says, "love thy neighbor as thyself." If you are not adequately loving yourself, then whatever you are doing for your neighbor is not being done out of genuine love, but some apparition of love and kindness. It reminds me of the times when I would go to the beauty shop to get my hair done, and I was always bothered by the hair stylist whose hair was in great disarray. It would be like going to an orthodontist who had crooked teeth. She was her own worst advertisement.

Now that you've made a time commitment to yourself, what are you going to do with that time? This would be a great opportunity to get in touch with your neglected side. There are things that have been in your heart, mind, dreams, and imagination that you've wanted to explore for so long. Now is the time to use all of your senses and do something new and wonderful. Maybe you should register for that class you always wanted to take. You could:

- sign up for karate lessons
- learn how to program your VCR and stop it from blinking 12:00
- start a vegetable garden
- take a belly-dancing class
- learn how to play the piano
- have a glamour-shot photo session
- join a travel club
- spend a weekend at a five-star hotel and order room service
- learn how to paint
- learn to sew, knit, do needlepoint, or crochet
- learn how to change a tire or do an oil change
- learn how to cook or bake
- take up a new sport
- start a collection
- write letters to loved ones on perfumed stationery, not e-mail
- buy lingerie for your own pleasure and wear it
- use your good china and crystal every day
- buy clothes that make you feel wonderful, not what others expect
- call up old friends
- ask someone you'd like to know out for dinner
- buy yourself flowers
- write yourself a letter, and tell yourself what you love about you

THE BETHANY HOUSE

Another life-nurturing activity women can cultivate is to be in relationships with friends that enhance their own *re-create-tion*. As children we used to spend at least four hours a day just playing. We had recess at noon and playtime after homework was finished. We played all day Saturday and on Sunday after church. When was the last time you played? Can't remember? I thought not. When you're planning your work, don't forget to plan your play.

There ought to be places where you can go and be renewed in the sensuous, loving spirit of friendship. We need to learn to seek intimacy through friendship. Jesus found this in the home of His friends Lazarus, Mary, and Martha. Theirs was a home where Jesus did not have to deal with the Pharisees and Sadducees, who were constantly testing Him and trying to find fault in His ministry and personal lifestyle. The Bethany House was a place where He could sit and talk, eat and laugh with like-minded men and women who allowed Him to be Himself. I've always pictured Jesus sitting at dinner with His friends, eating the first-century version of fried chicken, potato salad, greens (with hot sauce, of course), corn bread, peach cobbler, and sweet tea. No one constantly asking, "Jesus, what did the prophets mean when they said, 'blah, blah, blah.' " Some folks act as if they can't have fun unless they are in Bible study and prayer all the time. Relax. You ain't all that deep! Who would be more comfortable around you, the Pharisees or Jesus' crew? Yeah, that's what I thought. Again, the wisest man said, "There is a time and a purpose for everything." When was the last time you laughed, played a good game of bid whist, or danced? Try it. These are the kinds of relationships in which solid friendships are formed. The best intimacies in life are those conceived in friendship.

LAST THINGS . . .

The reality of life is this: Without love as the pure intention and motive of our actions and will, we are just going through the motions. Like mimes, we show no true feeling, have no meaningful expression on our face, and do not touch others around us. We are muted by the absence of love. Our heart is no more than a bit of red paint upon our shirt—it's not real. Unexpressed, our love has no dimensions, no depth, height, or width. We possess only a shallow substitute of the real thing. For we cannot truly love ourselves or our earthly companions because we have never truly loved our heavenly reality—God.

When we can humble ourselves and surrender our will to the will of a loving God, then we shall know love. This love is the life-giving force in the universe. This love is seen in the darkness of the night. It is heard in the silence of the early-morning dawn. This love informs our intellect, inspires our spirit, strengthens our body, infuses our heart, and clarifies our mind. A life separated from this love is a mere existence. The apostle Paul expressed it this way:

> If I speak in the tongues of mortals and of angels, but do not have love, I am a noisy gong or a clanging cymbal. And if I have prophetic powers, and understand all mysteries and all knowledge, and if I have all faith, so as to remove mountains, but do not have love, I am nothing. If I give away all my possessions, and if I hand over my body so that I may boast, but do not have love, I gain nothing. Love is patient; love is kind; love is not envious or boastful or arrogant or rude. It does not insist on its own way; it is not irritable or resentful; it does not rejoice in wrongdoing,

but rejoices in the truth. It bears all things, believes all things, hopes all things, endures all things. Love never ends. But as for prophecies, they will come to an end; as for tongues, they will cease; as for knowledge, it will come to an end. For we know only in part, and we prophesy only in part; but when the complete comes, the partial will come to an end. When I was a child, I spoke like a child, I thought like a child, I reasoned like a child; when I became an adult, I put an end to childish ways. For now we see in a mirror, dimly, but then we will see face to face. Now I know only in part; then I will know fully, even as I have been fully known. And now faith, hope, and love abide, these three; and the greatest of these is love (I Corinthians 13).

A new ethic, founded on the love of God, self, and neighbor, can be the beginning of something wonderful, powerful, and life-changing if you are willing to continually search your heart and have honest conversations about all aspects of your life. It is time for us to put aside childish ways, for they no longer serve us well. For we do know, in part, but we seek to walk daily with the One who makes all things new. "Beloved, we are God's children now; what we will be has not yet been revealed" . . . "But, as it is written, 'What no eye has seen, nor ear heard, nor the human heart conceived, what God has prepared for those who love him' " (I John 3:2, I Corinthians 2:9).

MY INWARD JOURNEY

Build a sacred space in your home for prayer, meditation, reflection, and soul nurturing. Place photos of loved ones there. Place a small waterfall that will provide the calming sounds of gurgling water (you can buy these in most department stores). If you cannot find one, place a bowl of water on your altar; water represents cleansing and healing. Place a candle or some incense upon the altar. Have nearby a musical instrument to play, or a bell to ring, or a music box. Drape a white fabric upon your altar and a symbol that brings to mind the presence of God's spirit. Then place something upon the altar that represents you as a woman, a daughter of the most high God.

Each person's daily devotion will look different. You may sing a favorite hymn or praise song. You may play a favorite CD (if others are near and you do not want to disturb them, use your headphones). Begin your meditation by "centering down." This is a time to become still, to enter into the re-creating silence, to allow the fragmentation of your mind to become centered. When meditating, there is an exercise called "palms down, palms up." You begin by placing your palms down on your lap as a symbolic indication of your desire to release any concerns you may have to God. Inwardly, you may pray, "Lord, I release to you my fear about next week's surgery. I give to you my anger toward Joseph. I surrender to you my anxiety about having enough money to pay the bills." Whatever it is that weighs on your spirit, just say "palms down." Release it. After several moments of surrender, turn your palms up as a symbol of your desire to receive from the Lord. You may silently pray, "Lord, I would like to receive your peace about next week's surgery, and your divine love for Joseph." Whatever you need, say "palms up." Having centered your mind and spirit, spend the remaining time in silence. Do not ask for anything. Allow the Lord to commune with you, to love you. If you receive some direction or communication from God, wonderful; if not, fine, just enjoy basking in the presence of your loving God.

"God always meets us where we are and slowly moves us along into deeper things."

—RICHARD J. FOSTER

"If you always do what you've always done, you'll always get what you always got—so do it differently."

Resources

What Works

The following is a partial list of church ministries designed to educate and serve the community in areas related to sex education,
health concerns, counseling, or problems related to family life. In
addition, a list of useful organizations is provided for further information, help, and guidance.

THE ARK OF REFUGE: HIV/AIDS MINISTRY
The City of Refuge United Church of Christ
1025 Howard Street
San Francisco, CA 94103
415-861-6130
www.arkofrefuge.org
Rev. Dr. Yvette Flunder, Founder and Senior Pastor

The City of Refuge United Church of Christ, founded in 1991, is a "radically inclusive" community built on the solid love that Jesus Christ has for all God's children. They believe there are no limits on the love of Christ and that everyone is worthy of God's love. City of Refuge welcomes people who come from all aspects of society, especially those who have felt shut out, isolated, and alone in their desire to be fully themselves and fully Christian. They welcome all people, saying, "We welcome you and all your baggage, for we are here, too, with all our baggage—working toward a personal and intimate relationship with God. City of Refuge/UCC is an open and affirming congregation, open and affirming to all those who have lost, left, or never had a church home. We welcome you, your children, your spouses, your partners, your parents, and all your relations, and hope you can find a church family here."

The Ark of Refuge is a ministry for promoting AIDS education throughout the African American community and in targeted high-risk groups. A component defining the program's uniqueness was and continues to be the "train the trainer" peer outreach to the religious and lay communities. The Ark of Refuge serves the underserved—people of color and women with HIV. Its programs expanded to include housing and direct services for low-income and homeless HIV-infected individuals through the creation of The Ark House, a communal living facility with comprehensive services, which is the first of its kind in Oakland.

Later, its programs expanded to include the multidenominational minister's Community Health Task Force, HIV-education training materials promoting ongoing AIDS/HIV education activities in the religious community, alongside the organization of a Women's Task Force on AIDS. This task force identified and trained church-based women as peer educators and group facilitators for workshops and seminars providing HIV education focused toward women at risk and their children.

During 1992, The Ark of Refuge, Inc., established Hazard-Ashley House for homeless HIV-positive men in Oakland, where they received comprehensive medical and psychosocial support services. In that same year, The Ark of Refuge, Inc., provided administrative and technical assistance to the Black Coalition on AIDS and Rafiki House, the first minority-operated HIV housing program in San Francisco. Restoration House, which opened in 1993, was a first-of-its-kind dual-diagnosis housing and substance-abuse treatment program for HIV-positive African American women in San Francisco. Residents there are provided with individualized substance-abuse recovery programs, along with coordinated HIV support services. Walker House was opened in 1994 as long-term supportive housing for low- or no-income people with HIV disease. At Walker House, services include nutrition management, coordinated medical and HIV support services, and a twenty-four-hour staffing pattern for medical emergencies and crisis intervention.

BALM IN GILEAD, INC.
130 West 42nd Street, Suite 1300
New York, NY 10036
212-730-7381
Pernessa C. Seele, Founder/CEO

The Balm in Gilead is a national, nonprofit organization founded in 1989 with its headquarters in New York City. Working through Black churches, the mission of the Balm in Gilead is to stop the spread of HIV/AIDS in the African American community and to support those infected with, and affected by,

HIV/AIDS. The organization seeks to accomplish its mission through the following programmatic goals:

- To build the capacity of Black church congregations to provide compassionate leadership in the prevention of HIV, to disseminate treatment information, and to deliver supportive services to those infected and affected in their respective communities.
- To build the capacity of community-based organizations and state and local agencies to collaborate effectively with Black churches to address the AIDS epidemic in the African American community.
- To raise awareness in the community at large of the Black church's unique strengths in facilitating the eradication of AIDS in the African American community and the need to support the church's development in this area.

The Balm in Gilead is recognized as one of the most effective and inspiring AIDS initiatives aimed at faith communities. It successfully engages denominational leaders, clergy, congregations, and individual parishioners in the AIDS struggle. The Balm in Gilead is the only AIDS service organization that has been endorsed by more than ten Black church denominations and caucuses. These endorsements provide the organization with the potential to bring AIDS prevention and treatment information to more than 20 million black Americans through their religious affiliations.

The Balm in Gilead provides churches with opportunities for training, networking, and education. Among these opportunities is the Black Church Week of Prayer for the Healing of AIDS, beginning the first Sunday in March of each year. This national initiative is an awareness program designed to bring African American churches into an effective dialogue concerning the issues of HIV and to act as a catalyst for the development of ongoing HIV programs. Another important component of the organization's efforts is the Black Church HIV/AIDS Resource/Information Center. The center produces educational and training products, including *The Black Church HIV Education and Prevention Guide* and *Who Will Break the Silence? Liturgical Resources for the Healing of AIDS.*

HIV/AIDS, SPIRITUAL, HEALTH AND WELLNESS CONFERENCE
Emmanuel Baptist Church
1 South Walnut Street
Colorado Springs, CO 80905
719-635-4865
Rev. Benjamin Reynolds, Pastor

Emmanuel Baptist Church sponsors an annual HIV/AIDS, Spiritual, Health and Wellness Conference. The goal of this mobilization, education, and risk intervention conference is to educate African American clergy, laypersons, and community leaders about resources, behaviors, and strategies to stop the devastation of the AIDS pandemic in the Colorado Springs community. The conference is designed to address problematic need factors such as culturally sensitive HIV/AIDS educational literature and information for use in the Colorado Springs African American community; to inform clergy, laypersons, and community leaders about local, state, and federal resources that will enable churches and community organizations to provide HIV/AIDS education, prevention, and risk reduction services to the communities they serve; and to train church leadership on how to develop community outreach programs.

The conference offers three intensive seminars for clergy and laypersons that offer training in HIV/AIDS education and prevention, training certification as part of the seminars, and culturally sensitive education materials for distribution to conference participants.

THE FLEMISTER HOUSE
527 West 22nd Street
New York, NY 10011
212-604-0124
Rev. Timothy Mitchell, Director
Flemister House is the American Baptist Churches of Metro New York City's hospice facility for people with AIDS.

THE LOVE CLINIC
214-922-0000
Fax: 214-922-0277
E-mail: revscp@theloveclinic.com
www.theloveclinic.com
Dr. Sheron C. Patterson, Founder
The Love Clinic is a faith-based, community- and relationship-building institute dedicated to healing hearts and homes in the Dallas/Ft. Worth area. This ministry was founded in 1995 by Dr. Sheron C. Patterson, a United Methodist pastor, who noticed increasing levels of social problems resulting from destructive relationships. Recognizing that God can help people free themselves of emotional bondage and break negative relationship patterns, she developed the Love Clinic to offer faith-related relationship solutions.

Their strategy is to present inspirational and informative

seminars on a wide range of topics, including, but not limited to, dating, marriage, and parenting at Dallas area churches; to host a citywide youth lock-in to educate and inspire youth in the areas of abstinence and developing healthy relationships; to host a three-session summer camp program for youth to teach them how to have healthy relationships with the opposite sex, their parents, and their siblings; to create and disseminate the Love Clinic Tour newsletter and the e-newsletter that offers relationship-building strategies and informs the potential Love Clinic attendees of up-coming events; to produce a celebration banquet to recognize the churches and youth who have participated in the Love Clinic Tour 2001; to sponsor a Love Clinic 5K Run to increase awareness of relationship issues in Dallas and raise funds for the Habitat for Humanity House.

THE BLACK CHURCH INITIATIVE OF THE RELIGIOUS COALITION FOR REPRODUCTIVE CHOICE

The Religious Coalition for Reproductive Choice
1025 Vermont Avenue NW, Suite 1130
Washington, DC 20005
202-628-7700
www.rcrc.org
Rev. Carlton W. Veazey, President and CEO

In 1997, the Religious Coalition for Reproductive Choice successfully launched The Black Church Initiative, a program to "break the silence" about sex and sexuality in African American churches. The initiative assists African American clergy and laity to address teenage pregnancy, sexuality education, and reproductive health within the context of African American religion and culture. The initiative consists of the following:

- The National Black Religious Summit on Sexuality
- Keeping It Real!: A faith-based model for Teen Dialogue on Sex and Sexuality
- Breaking the Silence: A faith-based model for Adult Congregational Dialogue on Sex and Sexuality

Keeping It Real! is a groundbreaking Christian sexuality education curriculum for African American youth. Developed by The Black Church Initiative of the Religious Coalition for Reproductive Choice, Keeping It Real! prepares youth to make healthy, responsible decisions as spiritual and sexual beings. The seven-week program of facilitated dialogue and activities is one of the first organized efforts in African American faith communities to address sex and sexuality in both a biblical and a secular context. African American educators and ministers now have a model to break the silence about sex and begin an open dialogue with youth. Keeping It Real! is for youth aged thirteen to seventeen. Youth meet in small groups of twelve to fifteen persons, with one clergyperson and one layperson to facilitate discussion. Designed for maximum participation, the sessions help enhance communication, cognitive, and reasoning skills through role plays, reading and active listening exercises, and interpretations of scripture and popular music and media.

THE UNITED CHURCH OF CHRIST
Justice and Witness Ministries
700 Prospect Avenue
Cleveland, OH 44115
216-736-2100
Ann L. Hanson, Minister for Children, Families and Human Sexuality Advocacy
For many years, the United Church of Christ has encouraged

churches and individuals to study the subject of human sexuality in their faith community and personally. We have published three resources for use in congregations: *Created in God's Image* (for older youth and adults), *Affirming Persons, Saving Lives* (for kindergarten through adult—HIV/Aids prevention focus), and our newest, *Our Whole Lives—Sexuality and Our Faith* (written in cooperation with the Unitarian Universalists).

For more than thirty years, the United Church of Christ has encouraged the study of human sexuality by local church members. In 1983, the General Synod of the United Church of Christ called upon the national setting of the church to develop resources for all ages on this subject, and age-span materials are now available for use. Our sexuality is an important part of being human and can be used to enhance our lives in ways that bring us closer to the Holy. However, because of fear, abuse, lack of education, or disease, it can be a cause of much pain and even death. The resources and ministry provided by the United Church of Christ help people of all ages to grow in their understanding that they are created in the image of God and that God's gift of human sexuality needs to be understood and celebrated. This belief is supported by our commitment to provide comprehensive resources that assist people in their decision-making processes.

PROJECT MIC
Holgate Street Church of Christ
2600 S. Holgate Street
Seattle, WA 98144
206-324-5530
James Hurd, Minister

Project MIC stands for Multi-Level Interfaith Church Domestic Violence Project. Located in Seattle, Washington, its mission is to educate church leaders of multicultural churches on domestic and youth violence, sexual assault, and substance-abuse prevention and awareness. It also provides effective responses to victims, survivors, and perpetrators of violence. The project's goals are to provide active and ongoing culturally sensitive support and follow-up responses to batterers in taking responsibility for violent behavior; to make the church a safe haven for victims and survivors of violence; and to provide safe, confidential, individualized support services and other resources.

Project MIC's services include individualized and group consultations for church leaders on effective responses to victim/survivors of violence and/or perpetrators; a clergy resource team of experts on these issues to provide information and support to church leaders; ongoing, beginning, and advanced-level training for ministers and other church leaders; and individual and group counseling for women, men, and teens.

For General Information

THE ASSOCIATION OF BLACK PSYCHOLOGISTS
P. O. Box 55999
Washington, DC 20040-5999
202-722-0808
E-mail: Admin@ABPsi.org

BLACK PSYCHIATRISTS OF AMERICA
2730 Adeline Street
Oakland, CA 94607
415-465-1800

THE NATIONAL ASSOCIATION OF BLACK SOCIAL WORKERS
15231 West McNichols Avenue
Detroit, MI 48235
313-836-0210

NATIONAL ASSOCIATION OF BLACK WOMEN
ATTORNEYS, INC.
724 9th Street, NW, Suite 206
Washington, DC 20001
202-637-4890

NATIONAL POLITICAL CONGRESS OF BLACK WOMEN, INC.
600 New Hampshire Avenue, Suite 1125
Washington, DC 20037
202-338-0800

NATIONAL COUNCIL OF NEGRO WOMEN, INC.
1001 G Street, NW, Suite 800
Washington, DC 20036
202-628-0015

NATIONAL BLACK WOMEN'S HEALTH PROJECT
1237 Ralph David Abernathy Boulevard, SW
Atlanta, GA 30310
404-758-9590

AIDS

NATIONAL HIV/AIDS HOTLINE
Centers for Disease Control
American Social Health Association
P. O. Box 13827
Research Triangle Park, NC 27709
800-342-AIDS
800-344-SIDA (Spanish)
800-243-7889 (TDD)

THE NAMES PROJECT—AIDS QUILT
800-872-6263

Sexual Abuse/Domestic Violence

THE BLACK CHURCH AND DOMESTIC VIOLENCE INSTITUTE
1292 Ralph David Abernathy Boulevard, Suite 100
Atlanta, GA 30310
404-758-0019
Fax: 404-758-9619
Rev. Aubra Love, Director

BLACK CHURCH AND DOMESTIC VIOLENCE INSTITUTE,
NORTHWEST

The Black Church and Domestic Violence Institute develops partnerships and collaborations to provide educational, spiritual, and technical support as well as advocacy and leadership development; to enhance the capacity of the church to empower and protect the victims of domestic violence; to hold abusers accountable; and to promote healing and wholeness in African American communities.

For more information:

Eleta Wright

425-259-2827

THE AFRICAN AMERICAN TASK FORCE AGAINST DOMESTIC AND
SEXUAL VIOLENCE

206-322-4856

www.aataskforce.homestead.com

Addresses domestic, dating, and sexual violence in the African American community.

SURVIVORS OF INCEST ANONYMOUS

World Service Office

P. O. Box 21817

Baltimore, MD 21222-6817

410-282-3400

INCEST SURVIVORS RESOURCE NETWORK

INTERNATIONAL, INC.

P. O. Box 7375

Las Cruces, NM 88006-7375

505-521-4260

(2–4 P.M./11 P.M.–Midnight EST)

THE NATIONAL SEXUAL ASSAULT HOTLINE

800-656-HOPE

TAMAR SPEAKS MINISTRY
Brooklyn, NY
718-771-0189
Dr. Valerie Andrews, Director

NATIONAL COUNCIL ON CHILD ABUSE & FAMILY VIOLENCE
1155 Connecticut Avenue, NW, Suite 400
Washington, DC 20036
800-222-2000
202-429-6695

THE NATIONAL DOMESTIC VIOLENCE HOTLINE
800-799-SAFE (7233)
800-787-3224 (TTY)

NATIONAL COALITION AGAINST DOMESTIC VIOLENCE
P. O. Box 34103
Washington, DC 20043-4103
202-544-7358

SEX EDUCATION AND PLANNING

THE SEXUALITY INFORMATION AND EDUCATION COUNCIL OF THE U.S. (SIECUS)
SIECUS Main Office
130 West 42nd Street, Suite 350
New York, NY 10036-7802
212-819-9770
Fax: 212-819-9776
E-mail: siecus@siecus.org

SIECUS is a national, nonprofit organization which affirms that sexuality is a natural and healthy part of living. Incorporated in 1964, SIECUS develops, collects, and disseminates information; promotes comprehensive education about sexuality; and advocates the right of individuals to make responsible sexual choices.

PLANNED PARENTHOOD FEDERATION OF AMERICA
810 Seventh Avenue
New York, NY 10019
800-669-0156
www.plannedparenthood.org
www.teenwire.com

Planned Parenthood affiliates operate 850 health centers nationwide. They provide medical services and sexuality education for millions of women, men, and teenagers each year—regardless of race, age, sexuality, disability, or income. They have many publications that are helpful in educating about sex, including *Having Your Period, How to Talk with Your Child About Sexuality, Human Sexuality: What Children Should Know and When They Should Know It, How to Be a Good Parent, Teensex? It's Okay to Say: No Way!, The Facts of Life: A Guide for Teens and Their Families, True Stories About Kids and AIDS*, and many more.

ADDICTIONS

NATIONAL COUNCIL ON SEXUAL ADDICTIONS AND COMPULSIVITY
1090 S. Northchase Parkway, Suite 200
South Marietta, GA 30067
770-989-9754

ALCOHOLICS ANONYMOUS (AA)
General Service Office
474 Riverside Drive
New York, NY 10115
212-870-3400

COCAINE ANONYMOUS
800-347-8998

NATIONAL COCAINE ABUSE HOTLINE
800-COCAINE

AL-ANON FAMILY HEADQUARTERS
200 Park Avenue South
New York, NY 10003
757-563-1600

CO-DEPENDENTS ANONYMOUS
602-277-7991

CHILDREN OF ALCOHOLICS FOUNDATION
33 West 60th Street, 5th Floor
New York, NY 10023
212-757-2100 ext. 6370
800-359-COAF

**NATIONAL ASSOCIATION OF CHILDREN OF ALCOHOLICS
(NACOA)**
11426 Rockville Pike, Suite 100
Rockville, MD 20852
301-468-0985
888-554-2627

WOMEN FOR SOBRIETY
800-333-1606

NICOTINE ANONYMOUS
2118 Greenwich Street
San Francisco, CA 94123
415-750-0328

OVEREATERS ANONYMOUS
National Office
P. O. Box 44020
Rio Rancho, NM 87174-4020
505-891-2664

GAMBLERS ANONYMOUS
National Council on Compulsive Gambling
444 West 59th Street, Room 1521
New York, NY 10019
212-903-4400

DEBTORS ANONYMOUS
General Service Office
P. O. Box 400, Grand Central Station
New York, NY 10163-0400
212-642-8220

Selected Bibliography

Brown Douglas, Kelly, *Sexuality and the Black Church*. (New York: Orbis Books, 1999.)

Foote, Catherine J., *Survivor Prayers: Talking with God About Childhood Sexual Abuse*. (Louisville: Westminster John Knox Press, 1994.)

Hollies, Linda H., *Taking Back My Yesterdays*. (Cleveland: Pilgrim Press, 1997.)

Moore, Thomas, *The Soul of Sex*. (New York: HarperCollins, 1998.)

Neiburg Terkel, Susan, *Finding Your Way: A Book About Sexual Ethics*. (Danbury: Franklin Watts, 1993.)

Weems, Renita, *Battered Love: Marriage, Sex, and Violence in the Hebrew Prophets*. (Minneapolis: Fortress Press, 1995.)

————, *I Asked for Intimacy: Stories of Blessings, Betrayals, and Birthings*. (Philadelphia: Innisfree Press, 1993.)

West, Traci C., *Wounds of the Spirit: Black Women, Violence, and Resistance Ethics.* (New York: New York University Press, 1999.)

Wyatt, Gail Elizabeth, *Stolen Women: Reclaiming Our Sexuality, Taking Back Our Lives.* (New York: John Wiley & Sons, 1997.)

ABOUT THE AUTHOR

The Reverend Dr. Susan Newman, an ordained minister for the past twenty-five years and a nationally recognized preacher/speaker, is the author of *With Heart and Hand: The Black Church Working to Save Black Children*. She makes her home in Washington, D.C.